MINDING
MUM

IT'S TIME TO TAKE CARE OF
YOU

ALISON CANAVA

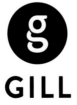

GILL

Gill Books
Hume Avenue
Park West
Dublin 12
www.gillbooks.ie

Gill Books is an imprint of M.H. Gill & Co.

978 07171 7028 9

Edited by Rachel Pierce at Verba Editing House
Designed by redrattledesign.com
Photography by Edina Valentova at Spirevision, assisted by Juraj Jabionka
Food and extra photography by Pearse Healy/Feena McCormack

Food charts on p.123 and p.126 courtesy of Liz Cook: www.lizcookcharts.co.uk
Illustrations by Storyboard Workshop
Food pyramid on p.128 illustrated by Derry Dillon
Printed by BZ Graf. S.A. Poland

This book is typeset in Archer.

The paper used in this book comes from the wood pulp of managed forests. For every
tree felled, at least one tree is planted, thereby renewing natural resources.

A CIP catalogue record for this book is available from the British Library.

5 4 3 2 1

This book is dedicated to an angel that was sent to me.
His name is James Joseph Canavan. He was born on
16 September 2010 in The Coombe Hospital in Dublin
and he saved my life.

Note from the Publisher

Information given in this book is not intended to be taken as a replacement for medical advice. Any person with a condition requiring medical attention should consult a qualified medical practitioner or therapist.

CONTENTS

INTRODUCTION: My Story So Far 1

CHAPTER 1:   What is Minding Mum? 17
CHAPTER 2:   Home Truths about the Early Days 29
CHAPTER 3:   Baby Blues and Post-natal Depression (PND) 55
CHAPTER 4:   Your Post-baby Body and Body Image 81
CHAPTER 5:   Nutrition 115
CHAPTER 6:   Exercise Post-pregnancy 185
CHAPTER 7:   Beauty Tips for Busy Mums 213
CHAPTER 8:   Mindfulness and Meditation 245
CHAPTER 9:   Stress and Work/Life Balance 265
CHAPTER 10:   The Art and the Importance of Gratitude 291

EPILOGUE   And the Story Goes On ... 303
A WORD OF THANKS 307

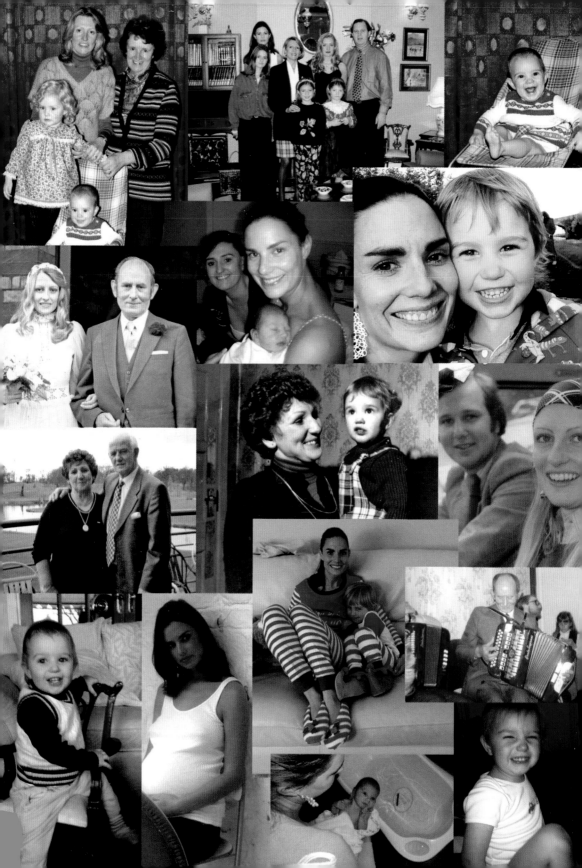

INTRODUCTION
MY STORY
SO FAR

What do we all want out of this life?

Well for me, I thought it would go something like this: grow up, get married, have a family. At least, that is how I wrote my original story. Not on paper, mind you, because there was really no need – how could the story turn out any other way? I'm a traditional girl at heart and simply love old school romance. I had visions of a house filled with laughter and life. My wedding would be big, but not ridiculous. We would have an old country-style house as well as our apartment in NYC, as that's where I lived. We would have the best of both worlds.

But sometimes life has a different plan and now I am writing this book in a park in Dublin instead of Central Park in New York. What brought me home was a very bright light called James. He is my son and my angel. His presence has taught me so much about life and what's really important. The past five years have been a rollercoaster ride of lessons and emotions. But really, all my life I've either been too high or too low and I have always craved consistency. I had lots of questions: does happiness exist, do I deserve it and, if so, how do I get there? I spent many years looking for answers to my questions, but it wasn't until I became a mum that I really started to work on myself and understand that the real beauty of life is what we have right now and that true happiness comes from within. The biggest lesson I have learned is that if you are not happy with what you have right now at this moment in time, you will never be happy, because what you want will keep tripping you up.

I'm incredibly analytical, which can be very annoying sometimes, and I discovered that at times you can question yourself into paralysis. The only way to be is to do, which is what I focus on now.

I grew up in a beautiful leafy suburb of Dublin called Castleknock, right beside the Phoenix Park. I'm the second eldest of five girls. My Mum was born in London, but her parents were Irish and my Dad was from Dublin. We were a typical family growing up. I played piano, violin and recorder. I did Irish dancing, ballet, tap and jazz. I sang in the school choir and I loved the variety of my life. I was always a bit dramatic and I remember many times my Dad telling me to 'save it for the stage'. When I announced I was giving up Irish dancing my teacher, Mrs O'Shea, was very disappointed and to be honest so was my Mum. Ever since that day Mum reminds me that all my classmates went on to be members of *Riverdance* and I could have been up on that stage with them.

I had itchy feet from an early age. I was a tomboy, adventurous, and I was always getting into strife. We had a huge green in front of our house where we played, with lots of trees to climb. I managed to get my head stuck in The Big Tree once and the fire brigade was called to cut me out! I was a risk-taker, a deep thinker; I did not conform and always challenged authority, including my parents.

But as I grew into my teens I spent many days and nights

searching for the meaning of life. I started to experience prolonged feelings of sadness. I wanted to sleep more and my interests in the things I once loved waned quickly. You might think, well it's normal for a teenager to want to sleep, but I now realise that this was different. Even though I wasn't unhappy, I thought it was completely normal to wake up every day and have to push yourself really hard throughout the day. I did this every day and I thought everyone else was doing the same. It wasn't until much later on, when I changed my lifestyle and got on top of my depression, that I realised there was nothing normal about it. As I wasn't unhappy as such and had a great childhood, these years were even more difficult because I felt ungrateful, confused, alone and quite tired at times. I remember my sisters saying to me in the mornings, 'Are you in a bad mood again?', but it wasn't really a bad mood it was just that I felt low because unless I was pushing myself really hard to be otherwise, that was simply how I felt.

I didn't tell anyone how I was feeling because I wasn't really sure myself. Like any teenager, I began to experiment and I now realise that this experimentation began a journey of self-medicating very early on in my life that continued for nearly 20 years. 'Party Ali' was born. I felt free, I felt good, I had confidence and I had no worries. I consistently and constantly tried everything down through the years in an effort to figure myself out. I had counselling, took medication, exercised like crazy at times, meditated (still do) and went on numerous retreats to 'find myself'. But while everything worked temporarily, I would still feel quite sad at times and I was simply unable to shake it off.

It wasn't until I began to recover from post-natal depression, after I had my son five years ago, that I decided once and for all I was going to get to the root cause of my problem. I changed my lifestyle completely and began to see and understand the power of good food, exercise and self-care. I attended a doctor called Dr Edmond O'Flaherty, who practices nutrient therapy, and he diagnosed me with Pyroluria. This is a genetic condition and essentially means that I have too many Kryptopyrroles in my blood/body and high levels of these bind to B6 and zinc, leaving them unavailable for my body to use. To put this in perspective for you: zinc is responsible for hundreds of biochemical functions in our bodies and B6, as well as playing an important role in energy and the central nervous system, also plays a part in the making of serotonin and, you guessed it, that's our happy hormone. Now, through supplementation and a good healthy lifestyle, my life is not a struggle at all anymore. I have finally realised that waking up and forcing yourself through your day is not normal.

At 15 years of age I entered the world of modelling and won a competition being run by the Irish TV show *Head to Toe*. After that, I got signed to Nevs Model Agency in London and Eddie Shanahan 'The Agency' in Dublin. The next year, in 1994, I went on to represent Ireland in the Ford Supermodel of the World competition in Las Vegas and the rest, as they say, is history. The top three girls went to New York and a few of us were handpicked for Paris, and I was one of those lucky girls. I flew to Paris straightaway after that competition and never looked back. I walked the runways for some of the biggest fashion houses in the world. I shot worldwide beauty campaigns and travelled to some breathtakingly beautiful places.

But if you are in any way lost and you enter my industry, it is very easy to get extremely lost within it. I was lucky to have a strong personality and family and friends who helped keep me grounded, but even still it was tough and it often felt like I was leading two different lives: schoolgirl, who had to buckle under expectations and 'behave'; and international model, who travelled during school holidays and for show season. There were some amazing older models in Dublin who were incredibly supportive, but there were some bitches, too, who liked running girls off runways and intimidating newbies. My first agent, Eddie Shanahan, is the best the industry in Ireland has ever seen. He was tough and had your back; you respected him and worked hard. Young girls need that in the modelling world as it can be a very difficult place to be.

I have lived all over the world, from Paris and London to New York and as far away as Sydney and Capetown. I took every opportunity to travel anywhere I could work and get an agency. It was exhilarating and exciting. I really was living the dream. But no matter where I went or who I was with, I couldn't shake off my periods of sadness. I felt angry and ungrateful and spent years beating myself up, and as a result of this I didn't always treat myself very well. My saving grace in the early years was my Dad. He was pretty clued in and he could see the self-destruct button I was pressing, so he kept an eye on me. No matter how far away I was, I always felt he could fix any problem I had, like a superhero. I rang him from Greece, once, in floods of tears after a precarious incident with a photographer and he had me on the next flight out of there.

When I was just 21 I lost my Dad to cancer and it was a huge loss to my entire family. He had only just turned 48 and Mum was left with five children. My sister Laura was doing her Leaving Certificate and my baby sisters, Grace and Kate, were only 11 and 12 years old. My sister Jennifer is a year older than me and she worked for my dad, so her pain of seeing an empty office every day is something that I just cannot imagine; it must have been unbearable. It hit us all very hard. My Dad's parents were also still young and losing a child very simply goes against the natural order of things. Dad has three wonderful brothers, too, but none of us has ever really been the same since.

I never wanted to worry Mum when I was away working and if I had felt lonely before, I felt much worse after my dad was gone. My Dad was tough, though, and down through the years when I came home crying because of bullies, he encouraged me to stand up to them and toughen up. Underneath it all he was both proud of and worried about me. In his final days in Blackrock Clinic the nurses told me how proud he was. I bought him a teddy and a card and when I visited it was in the cupboard, but the nurses told me that when I left he would take it out and show it to everyone. It was these little things that I clung to when he was gone. On his deathbed he asked me to stop smoking and go back to college as he worried about life after modelling. I stopped smoking for a while after that and threw myself into work and then did what he asked and returned to college to study marketing. I haven't left college since! I don't think I ever grieved my Dad properly. I didn't really know how to, so I stopped that pain by leaving once again and returning to my party lifestyle.

Life moved on and work was better than ever, but my periods of sadness became more prolonged and a few years later I lost the love of my life in London because I simply could not communicate my real feelings to him. It sounds strange, but I felt completely trapped in my own body, unable to piece together the sentences to express how I felt or indeed to ask for help. He would ask how I was but nothing would come out, I just could not speak aloud the inner conversation. Eventually, we went our separate ways. It was incredibly upsetting to watch someone I loved so much drift away from me. I will never forget the pain I felt when we broke up.

I lost a little piece of my heart that day, but again I did something I was very good at: I ran away.

There's no city quite like New York to take your mind off things. It was a fresh start, a new beginning. There's no denying that throughout my life I have always pushed myself, even during my darkest days. I pushed myself harder than ever in New York, but it also became easier to escape there than anywhere I had ever been before. This was amazing initially, but incredibly lonely as time went on. I was so lonely at times that even if I was exhausted, I went out just so I could have some company. I did meet some truly incredible people there, however, and some great teachers along the way. New York City ingrained in me the power of positivity and resilience. I learned to never give up, no matter how hard things got and, most importantly, I learned to dream big.

Towards the end of my life in New York I became frustrated that I hadn't found 'happiness' yet and I simply could not understand why. After all, I was living a life everyone dreamed about: there were no rules and no routines and every day was different and exciting. But I still had a huge void within me that I could not fill. I was frustrated because I was constantly being told how lucky I was. 'Do you know how many girls would love to be in your shoes, Alison?' 'You seem very ungrateful, Alison.' 'No matter how much someone does for you it's never enough.' 'Why are you so quiet, you would think with the life you have you would be happier?' Or the passive-aggressive versions of the same thing: 'You are so lucky, I wish I was like you'; 'I wish I had your life, some people have it all'; 'Imagine being born like you, my life would be a breeze'.

I now realise that as a result of these conflicting messages I lost my real voice very early on. I had insecurities, like every other young girl, but everywhere I turned I was being told they were not valid. I didn't know how to move forward, but I also knew I couldn't go back. Sometimes I felt I didn't fit in. Fashion wasn't my passion and I began to yearn for a simpler life. I longed for stability, love and security. My itchy feet were fast and they had enabled me to run all the time, to different cities, away from heartache and, most importantly, away from myself. However, none of this movement had filled the void or stopped the pain I was feeling. Happiness was a slippery adversary and it seemed every time I got close to it, it went further away. Quite frankly, I was finding the whole process exhausting.

I had read every self-help book known to man – in fact, if you had entered my New York apartment and looked at the shelf, you would probably have made your excuses and left! I went on crazy retreats with crazy people. I visited many different therapists and even acquired new problems I wasn't aware I had. Not one person during this time ever mentioned the words depression or anxiety. I had no idea that I had been suffering from depression and I now know this had started well before my life as a model. Despite not being treated for depression, I was given prescriptions early on for my symptoms. I took Xanax for air travel and Valium to sleep. I dipped in and out of antidepressants, but I was told they were just to help me cope with everyday life. Again, no mention of depression. Whenever I felt an emotion, I swallowed it with a pill. In fact, even the birth control pill was blamed for my low moods once and I was taken off it. I also drank my emotions and had smoked since my teens. I'm truly blessed with my genes because very early on I started to eat my feelings, too. I worked hard at drinking and became so good at it that I was always the life and soul of the party. I had loads of friends and I was invited somewhere every night of the week. I needed the highs and escapism to be higher, but in turn the lows became lower.

During these years I tried desperately to find a balance. I wanted to be like everyone else so I mimicked them. I didn't have a nine-to-five job but I decided to act like I did. I got up at the same time every morning and went to the gym. I tried every diet I came across and my life became a constant battle of trying to do the right thing while at the same time feeling like I was denying myself everything that gave me pleasure. I had rules, like only drinking at weekends, and I even gave up alcohol many times in an attempt to prove a point. I needed to prove to both myself and to others that my drinking habits were not an issue and were completely acceptable. I received mixed messages from friends and family and boyfriends who would remark about my lifestyle and then, when it suited them, pour shots down my neck because they wanted to party themselves.

During my time in New York I met a man, fell in love, had my heart broken and returned to Dublin in January 2010 to heal. It was a very difficult time in my life and I needed to be near my family and friends. We always imagine how we'd react in certain situations, but really it's not until we're there that we know. I hadn't been feeling well at all and I was exhausted, but I put it all down to the break-up. When I discovered I was pregnant, my mum and I cried for so many reasons. My family was always worried about my fertility because I had polycystic ovaries and had precancerous cells in my teens and twenties, but they knew how badly I wanted children. My situation was not ideal, however, and if I thought I had problems before, I really had no idea what lay ahead. I was in my third month of pregnancy when I found out. I was still taking the daily contraceptive pill and so now instead of worrying about it not working (which it clearly didn't), I was worried that it could have harmed my baby. Up until about 20 weeks I was horribly sick.

Everything made me sick, smells, cooking, rubbish, smoke – you name it, I couldn't handle it.

It became clear quite quickly that I was going to become a single mother; one of those women people gossiped about and judged. I didn't even have to look far for the inevitable as members of my own family kicked off the judgemental proceedings. There were also comments from strangers and to this day I thank all those people because they gave me the determination to fight. As I'm a glass half-full person, my sole focus was my health and wellbeing. This is where all my self-help and psychology books came into play. I believe in energy and that we are all made of energy and light. I simply had to make sure that I worked as hard as I could to prevent my baby from any negative energies and stress. I ate well, meditated, went for counselling and exercised; in fact, I don't think I had ever been as healthy as during my pregnancy.

My baby was born on 16 September at 11:43am. I called him James after my Mum's father, James Joseph. My Granddad was an extraordinary man who was the single biggest influence on my life as a child. I reckoned that if I could instil even some of his qualities into my James, he would be doing well. Granddad was kind, patient and very gentle. Mum's parents lived in London and when Granddad had a stroke I used to go over and visit him with Mum. Granddad was paralysed and had lost his speech, but he could say one word: Alison. I remember Granny asking why he couldn't say her name, and I still have a little giggle about that. Almost like our little secret. I had a connection to my grandfather like no other. I was only eleven then, but I spoke to him all the time. I spent hours talking to him and I always knew he could hear me, even if he couldn't respond. Even that day when I got my head stuck in The Big Tree, it was Granddad who had stood up for me, saying, 'Sure she's only a child, leave her alone'. I felt he really understood me, which is not something you can say very often in life.

I have always adored children and my friends and family often used to say that I had missed my calling and should be working with kids. At family gatherings or at friends' houses I always looked after the kiddies. I loved it so much that, to be honest, I wasn't too worried about becoming a mum. My main worries were being able to provide for James and give him the life he deserved. Modelling full-time abroad is very lucrative, but at home in Ireland there is limited work and I also had to face the reality that I wasn't 21 anymore. I needed to reinvent myself – but how? I was really lucky that during my pregnancy I became the face of Mothercare and did a pregnancy series for *Ireland AM* and shoots for lots of parenting magazines both in London and in Dublin. Post-pregnancy I began writing a column for *VIP magazine* and I loved it. I had a teacher who had always told me I was terrible at English and any time I was asked to write something, I would make my excuses. My editor at the time, Elaine Prendeville, gave me incredible encouragement and it was a real life lesson to learn to push through my fears.

I pushed myself way too hard, though, and returned to work just 10 days after giving birth to James. I felt I had no choice because as a single mum with no maternity benefit, I was worried about the basics, like buying clothes and food. I loved being a mum, but I found it really hard and I was tired all the time. I struggled to breastfeed James as he was tongue-tied and couldn't latch on properly. Eventually, with help from an amazing lactation consultant, Caitriona McCarthy, and my friend Andrea, I began to breastfeed successfully, albeit weeks after James was born.

I have always been teased for being too thin, so I presumed the baby weight would drop off quite easily. A part of it did drop off quite quickly, but then I really struggled with the rest. As my income and job depended on my body size and looks, I felt the pressure even more. I worked out really hard with a personal trainer, which was insane as afterwards I used to pull the car over on the way home and throw up. I was breastfeeding, and I remember often holding my swollen boobs and vomiting and cursing my career choice. My body also felt different and my shape had changed: having been a model for over half my life and being only 32 years of age, I really struggled with this. At the time my idea of a healthy lifestyle was quite warped anyway and I started to fall back into old habits of being really good for a week and then self-sabotaging and eating junk food to fill a void.

I continued on this crazy path, but to the casual eye I was Superwoman. No one could quite believe how well I was doing, including me. But as the weeks went on the simple everyday things became more and more difficult, until one day my world came crashing down. I was suffering from really bad post-natal depression and I needed help. However, this was the first time in my life I couldn't run away. I had to stand still and face my fears and my problems. It wasn't just about me anymore, I had James to think about. I became angry and frustrated because it is very painful to look within and work on yourself. I was given antidepressants that I really did not want to take as I was breastfeeding and because I was given no other option, this became a big turning-point in my life. I knew there had to be more to it than tablets. I attended counselling sessions, which I still do today if I need it, and I slowly worked through my pain. I read everything I could about depression and post-natal depression. I began to look at my lifestyle. I cleaned up my diet, exercised, meditated consistently and eventually weaned myself off medication. I began to understand the power of everything I was doing and over time I began to notice that I had discovered a formula and that it was working.

What I have learned is that even though I thought I had nothing when James was born because I was broke, worried and pretty terrified about the future, I actually had everything I needed. Five years on from that moment, I have learned so much about life and about myself. I have learned how resilient human beings are when the chips are down but, more importantly, I have learned that we always have choices, no matter how dark and difficult they might seem.

There were days when I thought I would never get a break, but my years in New York taught me to never give up and that voice in my head kept persisting, telling me that hard work does pay off. But when? I kept asking myself this because the waiting felt like torture. Every day I woke, put a smile on my face and pushed myself harder than ever before. There were just so many days when it got me nowhere, and it's so hard to keep the faith when life feels like that.

Sometimes I wanted to run before I could walk, but looking back I now realise that I was, and still am, moving at a pace that gave me the ability to grow into the person I have become today. I have learned to see the miracles in everyday life. I have finally learned to like myself, hell, even love myself after 37 years. Giving myself permission to do this has made a remarkable difference in my recovery from depression and anxiety. I have made changes to my life, very slowly, that have now replaced the old habits I used to fall into that were so destructive to myself, my family and my health and wellbeing. At times it seems to be a very hard and arduous road but let me tell you, it has been so worthwhile.

We are all born with the complete set of our own jigsaw puzzle, but it's how we put our jigsaw pieces together that makes the difference. Some people start with the borders and fill it to the centre; some people start with the corners and fit each piece onto it until it's done. That's the magic of life: we are all different and will deal with life and all it throws at us in our own way. I lost some key pieces of my jigsaw along the way, but eventually I found them again. We make our jigsaws at our own pace and that's okay too.

For years I searched for happiness to fill the gaping hole inside me. I always thought that the next job/party/boyfriend/holiday would do the trick, but now I know I have to look within as everything I need is already there. I filled the empty space through the years with parties and alcohol, I was in pain and that was my pain relief.

I now have a beautiful son and I give thanks every day for him because he saved my life. I'm dreaming bigger and living a better life than ever before. I never thought I would be able to tell my story, I never thought I could go back and study again, I never thought I would be good enough to rear James on my own and I never thought I could achieve being happy. But each day I'm achieving these things and more, and you can too. Sometimes, as mums, we think it's selfish to think of ourselves but I think it's selfless and that it's important to give yourself the permission to like and even love yourself, especially after a baby. Experiment and find your happy living formula, eat well and exercise, try some mindfulness or meditation and take time for yourself. Life can be hard work, but my advice is to work hard on the positive things that will make you healthy and happy rather than on the negative lifestyle habits that make life harder. It's up to you which life you choose.

During my recovery I was sitting on my single bed in Mum's house, where I was living at the time, and as I sat there I felt like a massive weight had been lifted off my shoulders. It was the first time I genuinely felt free and content. I had never had less but I had also never had more, and I wanted to figure out how to hold onto that feeling forever. Happiness is not a normal state to be in all the time and I have learned that being in a place of contentment is a more realistic aim. I have learned to manage myself and my time better, I do what's important to me, I have finally found a balance and I'm chasing my dreams. It's important, even as a mum, to chase your own personal dreams, no matter what anyone tells you. Five years ago I was pregnant with my first child, I was absolutely terrified and all I saw were broken dreams, but now I have assembled the missing pieces of my jigsaw. You can do it, too. We are all capable of so much more than we imagine and so much more than we think we deserve.

When I spoke out publicly about my depression, I was overwhelmed with support from other mums. To this day whenever I feel like giving up, an e-mail always seems to pop into my inbox at the right time from a mum who is struggling and who finds my outlook on life and my writing an inspiration. Sometimes women can be very unsupportive of each other, I've learned that the hard way, but it's the support of other mums in Ireland that carried me through the toughest time of my life, and for that I am very grateful.

This book is for all of you x

Alison

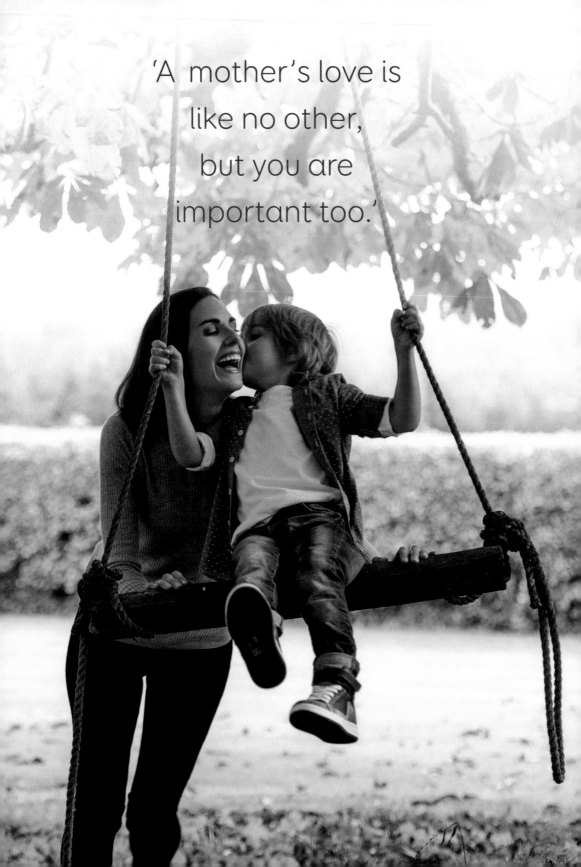

'A mother's love is
like no other,
but you are
important too.'

WHAT IS MINDING MUM?

I spent my pregnancy trying to adjust to the idea of being a single mum, or should I say attempting to accept the fact that things had turned out quite differently from how I had imagined they would be. The early days were tough and looking back now, I can't quite believe the pressure I put myself under. I was in a blind panic from the minute I gave birth. I was broke, living with my mum and I felt this overwhelming sense of responsibility for this little person who had just been born. I remember one evening when he had fallen asleep in his Moses basket and I thought, I'll just pop out for some milk. It was like a lightning bolt when I realised I could never go anywhere without someone looking after James … *ever again*. Now you might think that this is ridiculous, but I had never really thought about that part during my pregnancy. I suddenly felt this overwhelming sense of responsibility and if I was panicked before, I was even more panicked now!

I also remember trying to pack up the car to head out for an hour. Every time I left, half the house came with me and yet I always seemed to forget something. One morning as I was packing up the car, I was secretly delighted with myself as this time I knew I had everything. I hopped in the car and turned to check on James, but he wasn't there! In my effort to remember everything I had forgotten the most important thing of all. Luckily, I was only a few hundred metres away and when I opened the front door my little angel was sitting in his car seat, blissfully unaware of what had just happened. I told him that Mummy had forgotten him but not to worry – as he was so young there would be no lasting emotional damage for him, just for me!

As time went on I remember thinking how little I had been told about the reality of being a new mum. Throughout the western world we prepare mums very well for pregnancy and for the birth, but we completely forget about them post baby. When the baby arrives, nearly all new mums tend to neglect themselves because all the focus is on this precious new bundle. As you can see from my own story, I was so busy obsessing about things that I personally never came into the equation.

When you have a new baby lots of people come to see the baby, they buy gifts for the baby, they want to hold the baby, kiss the baby and are deeply concerned about the baby – but what about you? I remember Mum's friend, Margaret, and one of my own friends, Andrea, bought me a gift for myself and I cried. My reaction was: *For me, really? No, I can't take it. I'll feel bad.* But I was so touched that someone had thought of me.

Why is it that we seem to respect ourselves much more when a baby is growing inside us? During our pregnancy we are encouraged to mind ourselves all the time by eating well and exercising. During pregnancy, relaxation and time out is not a treat but a necessity, whereas afterwards it's a sin. We are monitored and cared for by doctors, midwives and nurses. Everywhere you go people look at your belly and ask how you are. People mind you and make a fuss of you and, let's be honest, it makes you feel very special. But what happens after the baby is born?

From the moment we give birth we feel guilty. We skip meals, have sleepless nights, we worry about everything and everyone but ourselves. We feel like a stranger in this new body. We're not sure how to dress it or how we feel about it and although we do know that we have just given birth, we can still feel insecure and emotional.

During my Mum's time women were allowed to stay in hospital for up to five days, now you are lucky if you get to stay in for 48 hours. I'm one of five girls and Mum said the more children she had, the more precious and important those five days in hospital became to her.

If the world was a DVD player, I would have sent it in to be repaired years ago because the Fast-Forward button appears to have got stuck. In fact, it seems to be getting faster and faster every year. Medicine and technology have advanced at an alarming rate, but our basic human needs remain the same, no matter how fast things go. We need to feel safe, loved and have good physical and mental health and, in my opinion, a woman needs all of this and more after a baby because you are more vulnerable than ever. You need time with your baby and time to recover post-birth and these are two things our fast-paced world won't allow.

If you ask any mother what 'minding Mum' means, they will probably laugh at you. The question would be met with a mixture of nervous laughter and probably some confusion as they ask: *'Mind me? Are you joking? I can't even go to the toilet by myself these days.'* But what starts off as a joke can turn into something more serious for a lot of women. Minding Mum is something very few women do after they have a baby, for so many reasons.

But what is so wrong with mums minding themselves and why do we feel so guilty about absolutely everything? We can be our own worst enemies, always judging each other and ourselves and, I'm sorry ladies, but it's time to wake up. As women we need support and solidarity, not judgement and harsh comments. Women are amazing and when we work together and support each other, there is nothing we can't do.

The idea for minding mum came to me primarily because I needed minding myself and because when I was touring around Ireland with my original 0 to Toddler shows, what struck me were all the questions and e-mails I received from mums who, just like me, felt lost and lonely. They felt they had lost their identity and their confidence and they were insecure in their new body and in their new role as a mum. There was a constant nagging feeling that they weren't good enough and probably never would be. They had lost the ability to trust themselves and their own decisions and without it they were guilty and flailing.

So let's think about this then: what really changes when we have a baby? Of course we need to look after the baby, but what do we need as mums to look after ourselves? And what does our baby need from us post-birth?

For me, the answer to both of these questions is simple and the exact same: a healthy, strong, happy Mum. Eureka! So why do we feel so bad about caring for ourselves when we become parents?

Why We Need To Mind Mum

As mothers we owe it to ourselves and our families to take care of ourselves for many reasons:

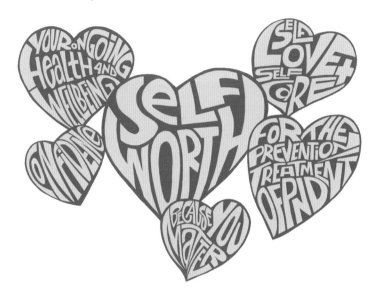

I was facing all these questions after James was born, so I set off on a journey of discovery. I was fascinated by this 'mummy club' that seemed to hold onto all these secrets and not let them go until you enter the club, by giving birth, at which point every mum on the planet suddenly becomes happy to share every tiny, awful detail with you. I remember being in a mum and baby group where all the mums were talking about how amazing their babies were – they were sleeping through the night, so advanced for their age – and I felt completely inferior by comparison. When I said that my baby wasn't sleeping through the night and wasn't feeding that well, some of the mums quietly admitted that theirs weren't either. So there you have it, no one says a word to you until you speak out and tell the truth. But why is this?

For some reason we seem to think that if we tell other women the truth, it will put them off becoming a mum. As a result, there is a chorus of mother talk that says only positive things, airbrushing out the harder parts. It would be far, far more helpful if we all – women, pregnant women, mums – spoke honestly and openly about the issues because that would prepare the newcomers, inform women in making decisions about having a family and help all mums to feel less lonely and more in control. It would make things a hell of a lot easier. I wish someone had been honest with me about the reality of breastfeeding and the possibility of post-natal depression. If I had known that 60–70% of women suffer from the baby blues, I wouldn't have felt like such a failure when I was crying alone a few days after the birth and feeling like the only mum in the world who couldn't cope (see Chapter 3).

> *It's simple: you need a little of everything and not a lot of one thing.*

So that was how it all began. It struck me that there was a wide gap between what women were saying and how they appeared, and what was going on behind-the-scenes in their daily lives. The more I write and the more I speak and the more I talk honestly to other women, the more I see just how much mums neglect themselves, almost sacrificing themselves for their families. This was why I decided to start a series of *Minding Mum* talks, to broach this emotional subject and get women talking about it. After all, there is no point in putting on make-up and nice clothes if you are crying inside.

In life we tend to focus on one area at a time, such as our diet, thinking that if we get it right, then we can move on to the next thing – maybe exercise or further education. I used to meditate once a week in New York and I would feel great afterwards, but soon the feeling would subside until the next week when I did it again. When

I took up a new exercise I would give it my all, training six or seven days a week. When I got bored with that, I would embark on a new diet. All of these things gave me temporary fixes, but I needed a permanent solution to my problems. The truth is that everything needs to work together, synergistically, for real change to happen. There are lots of options to choose from, so have fun finding a formula that works for you.

Find Your Formula

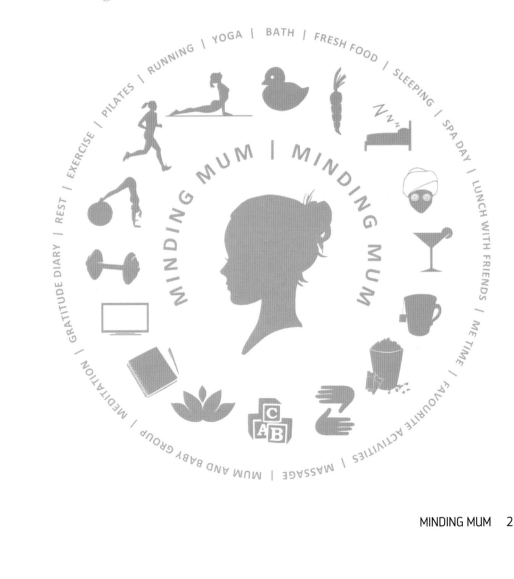

Your formula will change at different times in your life. What you need today or tomorrow will be different next year. When you are pregnant you will have a formula to suit, but it will change when the baby is born and you become a new mum. Have fun with it and try new things. But always remember that life is for living, so do what you love and not what you dread. Don't go to the gym if you hate it; try other types of exercise instead, like cycling or yoga. Never diet, just eat simple fresh food that tastes good. Finding your best formula can be frustrating, but it can also be a lot of fun.

After my post-natal depression I rebuilt my confidence slowly and realised how amazing we are as women and what a miracle it is to give birth. I have learned to love and respect myself much more than ever before, but that has taken hard work and time. On this journey I really began to understand the connection between body and mind. I had been treating them separately for so long, but really they are one. I had always treated my symptoms but never the cause.

When I started to treat my body better, by nourishing it with good food, my brain began to thank me by lifting my depression. I found an exercise routine I liked and wrote a gratitude diary every day. I went for counselling and meditated, but for me the most important part of all was that I decided it was okay to like myself. Once all of these jigsaw pieces started to fit together, the power of the 'big picture' was immense.

Small changes over time can make a big difference. They add up to a permanent lifestyle change and let me tell you that when you start to feel good, sleep well and have more energy than ever before, you will never look back. If Mum is not happy and healthy, it creates a domino effect within the family. That is why we need to focus more on mums and not solely on the baby because if Mum is healthy and happy, then you can be sure her baby is being taken care of very well.

I very often hear women say that when they have kids their life will be complete and if I'm honest, I thought this myself once. But our children should be adding something to our lives and not replacing something that's missing, which is why it's vitally important that we retain who we are after we have children. In my opinion we don't own our children, we are lent them for a short time until they blossom and grow into adults and make their own decisions, then the cycle will continue again. The thing is, though, we don't want to lose ourselves during this journey.

It can be very easy to get lost in our children, like a refuge from reality or from the real you. You can hide from yourself and always talk about the children, but this can be dangerous and tends to lead to confidence issues and self-worth problems. Doing things for yourself and keeping your own interests alive is incredibly important.

> " *Sometimes women start to question their abilities as an individual and 'Mum' ends up being the only thing they are – everything else gets jettisoned.* "

We all want happiness for our children, so turn that feeling back on yourself, look inwards and really start wanting it for yourself. There are many ways to do this. Being present in the moment is probably the most powerful and important way, but often the most difficult for most of us (see Chapter 8). We can also focus on being grateful for what we have right here and now because if we don't appreciate what we have now, we will never be happy with more (see Chapter 10). Sometimes we can't control what happens to us, but what we can control are the choices we make moving forward. As a mum I believe you need to mind yourself and be content. If you want to work, work; if you want to stay at home, then stay at home; no one has the right to judge you either way. What works for one person doesn't work for another. My work keeps me alive and I'm a happier person and a better mother because of that. I choose to work hard and study to provide for James in the best way I can. There are times I wish I had more time at home, but my golden rule is to be fully present when in his presence.

In this book I'm going to share with you some of the *Minding Mum* tips and tricks I've picked up along the way. We will look at the reality of the celebrity post-birth body and how it affects our own body image. I will share some beauty tips I picked up during my years in the fashion industry. We will look at the importance of good food for our bodies now and in the future. We'll be discussing how to enjoy your kids, worry less, use your time better and, most importantly, what gratitude means. In doing all this, the aim is to build your confidence as a new mum, which will help you to follow your dreams, big and small. This book is about joining the dots and living a better life for you and your family.

Minding Mum is about making the choices that suit you, that make you happy, that make you feel good. *Minding Mum* is about nurturing your inner beauty and letting it shine through. Let's move on from feeling bad and sacrificing ourselves for others and let's change the way we think about mums. We love our children unconditionally and many of us willingly give up so much for our children. My plea in this book is that you not let self-care become one of those sacrifices.

Remember, the best mums put themselves first!

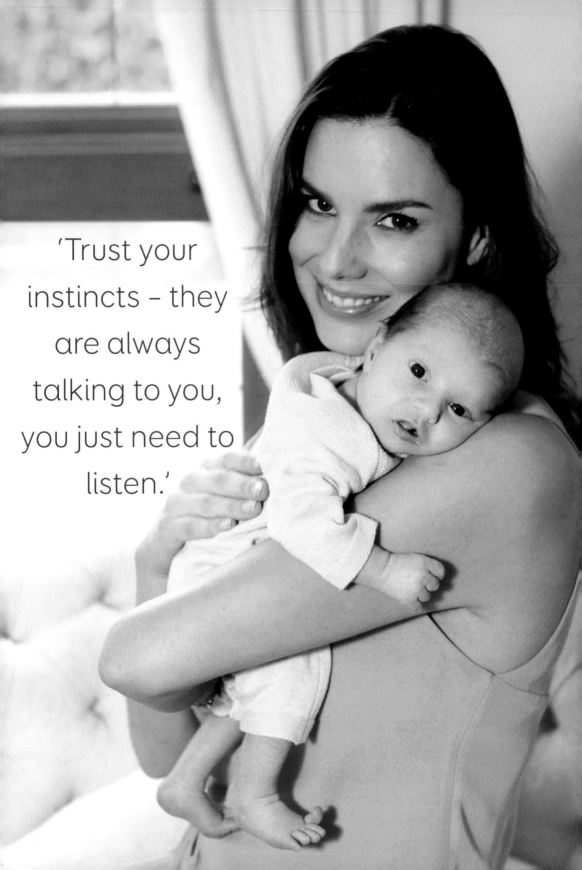

'Trust your instincts – they are always talking to you, you just need to listen.'

HOME TRUTHS ABOUT THE EARLY DAYS

2

When you are facing into becoming a parent for the first time, it's quite likely you'll feel thrilled and terrified all at once. There is the birth to get through, but after that things get a bit hazy and you're unsure how you'll cope, what you'll need and how you should prepare. As a soldier on the frontline, I'm going to radio back some hard-earned advice on what the early days are really like and how best to ready yourself for them.

All Brand new

There is absolutely no way of knowing how you will feel and think once your long-awaited baby arrives. After nine months of being a pregnant woman, being a mum is a completely new challange. The important thing is not to be scared or guilty about your emotions – they might well be topsy-turvy and unpredictable in the early days.

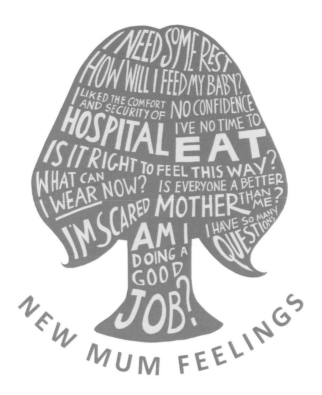

The important thing to remember about all of these questions and more is that they are completely natural and normal. Any time we experience change in our lives there is a readjustment period, and having a baby is no different.

Baby stuff

The first thing that will hit you when you become pregnant is advertising. You will be bombarded with advertisements of the latest 'must-have' products that you simply cannot raise a baby properly without. The latest, greatest buggy, car seat, cot and carrier all advance so quickly from one model to another, they put iPhones to shame. It's a world of built-in obsolescence and unending temptations designed to make you feel 'ready'.

Even though I have 22 years in the fashion industry under my belt, where I have always been selling some product or another, I'm ashamed to admit I am still a marketer's dream. When I first moved to New York I bought nearly everything that appeared on the infomercials on TV, until one day I realised that most of the products did not do what they promised and that my small apartment couldn't house us all happily.

Then my mother arrived for a visit and it was clear where I got my gullibility from: the first day I left her alone, I arrived home from work to my beaming mother who was bursting to show me the amazing products she had bought. 'You will never have to scrub again', 'Tess [my dog] will never get fleas or ticks' and 'now that you live in New York and space is limited, I have bought you storage bags that you hoover the air out of'. I must admit, a small part of me was excited too, but that summer Tess still got ticks and the bags kept filling with air after being sealed. I warned my mother off TV remote shopping and sent her back to the shops.

Even having gone through all this and believing myself to be smart about buying choices, when I got pregnant I still salivated over buggies that could practically take your kids out by themselves. Money was tight, but my kid deserved the best. After all it was my first child, I was about to become a single mum and what if I never had another baby ever again? To this day I still have unopened must-have products in my home, which begs the question: how on earth did my baby survive?

 Top tip

Babies do not need as much stuff as we think they do!

Breastfeeding

I was pretty terrified about labour and birth, but luckily it all went well. The first hurdle I encountered, therefore, was feeding. I didn't really think about which way I would feed my baby before I gave birth. Mum breastfed all of us and I've seen the beautiful movies of childbirth where baby pops out and immediately latches on to mum's breast, a bond is formed and all is good with the world. So while I didn't give it much thought, in the back of my mind I thought it would be just like that.

For me, feeding was the first frustration of motherhood. James could not sustain his latch and feed. I took to pumping and eventually the doctor realised that James was tongue-tied, which is when the string of tissue under the tongue (frenulum) that attaches the tongue to the floor of the mouth is too short. If your baby has tongue-tie, the tongue can't move freely and this can cause problems. As the tongue is one of the most important muscles for speech and swallowing, if this problem is not picked up early it can lead to eating or speech problems, which may be serious in some individuals. It's worth asking about it if you are having breastfeeding problems.

Even when we had figured out the cause, I still needed a lactation consultant to help me gain confidence with feeding. Every time someone latched him on for me he seemed to feed no problem and it looked quite easy; when they left me alone, I struggled really badly. I think this was a mixture of frustration, which the baby could obviously feel, and the fact that my confidence was very low at this stage, with a bit of impatience thrown in for good measure, too. I also developed nipple Thrush, which was incredibly painful. But I was lucky that I had a lot of milk, so pumping became my new pastime and soon there was a freezer full of milk. I eventually succeeded in feeding James, but I do remember thinking how great it would have been if someone had explained to me that sometimes feeding doesn't happen easily and naturally and can take time for both mum and baby to master.

One thing that can help this process is skin-to-skin contact. As soon as your baby is born, ask for skin-to-skin contact, or kangaroo care as it's better known Down Under. This is incredibly important and something I didn't know about when James was born, but from all my research I now believe it is an essential part of the birth process. It will help your baby recover from the birth, regulate your baby's temperature, glucose, metabolism and heart rate and enable your baby to hear your heartbeat, which is a comforting sound they have become accustomed to over the past nine months. It also helps both mum and baby to reach a more relaxed and calm state post-birth. We should never underestimate the power of touch. It's the first sense we acquire and the first language in which we become fluent. It gives us the ability to communicate non-verbally and makes our baby feel safe. Let's face it, who doesn't love a cuddle – even at our age! Finally, if you had a difficult birth or a Caesarean section, skin-to-skin contact will help you to bond with your baby. For all these reasons, make sure to ask your doctor or midwife to place the baby on your chest immediately after birth.[1]

If the birth has gone well and the baby is calm, babies will follow their own instincts and start to open their mouths, looking for food. Like all mammals, babies have an amazing sense of smell and will be able to locate the breast by following the smell of the

1 For more information on skin-to-skin go to: http://www.kangaroomothercare.com/index.htm; http://www.drjacknewman.com/. A couple of useful articles if you're interested: Dr Robin Grille, 'Attachment, the brain and human happiness'. GOLD Health e-learning conference 2010. Dr Jane Morton, 'Headaches in Breastfeeding Management'. GOLD Health e-learning conference 2010. Dr Nils Bergman, 'The scientific basis for Kangaroo Mother Care'. LLL national conference 2010.

colostrum, which has the same smell as the amniotic fluid they were swallowing in utero. The baby can also smell the amniotic fluid on his hands and since amniotic fluid is a pheromone (it has a smell and taste) and pheromones are specific to each mother and her breast milk, this helps to assure the baby that he is in the right place.

Top tip If you would like to try breastfeeding your baby, please ask for help if you need it. Inform yourself beforehand because as the saying goes, 'fail to prepare, prepare to fail'. If necessary, get a lactation consultant in to help you in the early days.

When things weren't going so well with James and I was feeling frustrated, I suffered an attack of Bold Child Syndrome (tell me not to do something and I will do it), which means I became obstinately determined to succeed. I began to educate myself about breastmilk and the reasons why it is considered the optimum form of feeding. The World Health Organization (WHO), for example, recommends breastfeeding exclusively for the first six months and to continue it through weaning for two full years. Similarly, the American Academy of Pediatrics (AAP) recommends breastfeeding for a minimum of 12 months, and for as long thereafter as baby and mother mutually desire. It's a completely personal choice, but if it is something you would like to try, give yourself the best chance of success by gathering all the information you need and accepting all the help that's offered. It might take some teeth-gritting to get through the early days, but remember that your body knows what to do and is capable of doing it.

James weaned himself and I did genuinely miss that connection as he grew. I now look at pictures of a breastfeeding mum and realise that it's the most natural thing in the world, even if it doesn't come naturally to all of us. I also had some breast milk in the freezer for nine months, which I used in his food and also gave him when he became ill.

When your baby teethes the analgesic (pain-relieving) properties that your breast milk contains will automatically increase. As a result, your baby will usually want to breastfeed more often when he is teething because it helps relieve pain and discomfort. How amazing are our bodies!

Top tip

Our bodies, the milk we make and how that milk is unique to each baby fascinates me. According to research done in Ireland in 2013, babies who are breastfed for three to six months are 38% less likely to be obese at nine years of age, while children who are breastfed for six months or more are 51% less likely to be obese at nine years of age. Breastfeeding also protects the baby from high cholesterol and diabetes in later life. There are great benefits for mums, too, according to La Leche League International, as breastfeeding can help prevent high blood pressure, heart disease and diabetes in later life and also ovarian and breast cancer (see *The Womanly Art of Breastfeeding,* La Leche League International).

One of the most important things I have learned as a mum is that your kids tune into your energy, so if you are stressed, panicked and upset, your baby will feel that. This is why I always say that how you choose to feed your baby is no one else's business. I have lots of friends who could not breastfeed for many different reasons and also through choice. I have also met many women who would have liked to breastfeed but found it too difficult and needed more support. We all have different reasons for feeding our children the way we do and it is important never to underestimate the complex issues that can arise post-birth for mum and baby and that can factor into and influence your feeding choice.

How you feed your child does not affect your parenting abilities. I have never quite understood what enrages women so much on this issue. If you feel you have made the correct decision, why would you feel the need to shout down the opposition? Every woman's story, and indeed journey, is unique and individual. My story began in ignorance, thinking baby comes out, latches on and we all live happily ever after. How wrong was I?

Whether you want to breastfeed or not, I do believe we are entitled to make informed decisions. In order to do that, we need information. I think that preparing mums for problems is incredibly important. It will equip you with skills and give you a better chance to succeed. It will also help you to realise that, whatever problem you encounter, you are not alone – lots of other women have been in your position before and many more will be in your position in the future.

The great rush of love

Every mum I speak to talks about the incredible love they feel for their children. My own mother used to say to me, 'you will never understand how worried I am about you until you have kids of your own'. This was said during my wild teenage years when I failed to understand why she stayed up waiting for me (I thought I was bulletproof during those years). But not long after James was born

I actually apologised to my mother for all the heartache and worry I had caused her down through the years because all of a sudden I completely understood what she meant.

I love James so much and honestly can't remember my life without him. Every day he makes me smile and I laugh all the time when I'm with him. I have to be honest, though: when he was born, I didn't feel an instant bond or connection with him. I never mentioned this to anyone because I felt so bad about it. When I was pregnant I truly felt that I would be a great mother, but then I thought there was something wrong with me because I didn't feel an overwhelming gush of instant love. It did come quickly enough, however, and continued to grow stronger each day. The day after he was born, on Friday, 17 September, I can remember thinking what an incredible feeling this was. He was so beautiful. On Saturday, 18 September I wrote in my diary: I'm really falling in love with him now.

As I became stronger as a mum and found my voice, I asked other mums about this and I was both comforted and surprised at all the mixed answers I received – no two answers were the same. One of my best friends said that she didn't gush with love straightaway. She said it was almost like the baby was a stranger for the first while. She was wrecked and had no energy and it took a few days for the love to kick in. She too felt relieved when she found out she wasn't the only one. Another friend was the complete opposite and felt an instant rush of love, describing it as overwhelming in a positive sense. Yet another friend told me that she was completely over the top with her daughter and almost too enamoured. She became incredibly nervous of anyone touching or feeding her baby and wouldn't leave her with anyone.

It's clear, then, that you can experience a whole range of emotions and feelings right after you give birth. The key is to recognise your emotions and feelings and not feel bad about them. Speak up and ask for help and tell someone how you are feeling, it will not be the first time they have heard it, you can be sure. The simple truth is that you just don't know how you are going to feel when your baby arrives, and the same goes for subsequent babies. Allow yourself to go with the flow as much as possible and if that gush of love doesn't happen instantly, don't worry, it just means you are living in the real world and not in Hollywood. Whatever happens, you are not alone – lots of other mums have felt that way, too.

How you will feel post-birth

Immediately after birth you need to start taking care of yourself. If you thought you needed pampering during your pregnancy, multiply that by a million because you will need lots of reassurance, cuddles and comfort. Rest when you can in the early days and sleep when the baby sleeps. This might only be a few minutes every day, but it's worth it. Obviously if you have more than one child this can be difficult, but you do need to do this to give your body and mind time to heal and recover. If possible, organise it so that you are relieved of all duties except feeding and caring for yourself and the baby. For now, just be a mum – you have plenty of years to be a house slave!

If you had a vaginal birth, you can expect to have some soreness for a few days and up to a few weeks after the birth. Some people have stitches or have undergone an episiotomy (a surgical cut to your perineum, which is the muscular area between your vagina and your anus) or, like me, you might have some lacerations. You may also have bruises from the pressure of the baby's head during birth.

*Here are some useful tips to help ease
discomfort post-birth:*

* take warm baths with salt (optional) to promote healing;

* do pelvic floor exercises as this will speed up recovery
  and improve blood flow to the area;

* use frozen peas or a frozen gel pack wrapped in a cloth on
  your perineum;

* pour lukewarm water over the area when urinating as this
  will help to reduce the stinging by diluting your urine;

* pat, don't rub, your stitches dry with toilet paper afterwards;

* sit on a ring or cushion if it's uncomfortable for you to sit
  after birth;

* to help with bowel movements, take a stool softener and
  drink plenty of prune juice (more on this in Chapter 5);

* keep very well hydrated;

* keep the area clean and shower often;

* have plenty of maternity pads and change them often.

Recovering after a C-section is different because you are recovering from major abdominal surgery. In this case you'll be looking at good pain relief, especially in the first few days as discomfort is common. You will also need to take good care of your incision and watch out for any signs of infection.

Here are some useful tips to help you recover from a C-section:

* rest whenever possible and try to have everything you need within reach to limit reaching and stretching;

* support your abdomen with your hand when you cough, sneeze or laugh;

* avoid lifting anything heavy (except for your baby, of course);

* seek pain relief, if necessary;

* gentle heat pads or a warm hot water bottle can help (see https://www.urmc.rochester.edu/ob-gyn/obstetrics/after-delivery/pain-management.aspx);

- keep hydrated for overall health, to prevent constipation and if breastfeeding;

- look out for signs of infection and contact your doctor if the incision is red, swollen or leaking discharge, if you have a high temperature or if the pain is increasing and not decreasing.

Post-pregnancy bleeding

No one told me about bleeding post-pregnancy and some of you might be thinking that it's basic common sense, but I had no idea of what was considered normal and what was not. When I got home from hospital and was dealing with things on my own, I found myself panicking when I had a sudden rush of blood and I felt insecure about calling the doctor, or indeed telling my Mum! Sometimes we get nervous, embarrassed and insecure about the silliest of things and that's okay too. So below are some guidelines for you regarding what's normal and what's not. Of course, if you are ever in doubt, do not hesitate to contact your GP or public health nurse.

What's normal?

Whether your birth was natural (vaginal) or via C-section, every single new mum will experience bleeding because this is how your body cleanses itself and gets rid of the lining of your womb (uterus) after the birth. This blood flow, which is called lochia, will be different for everyone. For some, the blood may come out in gushes, while for others it might flow more evenly, quite like a heavy period.

Some mums find that when they return from hospital their bleeding becomes heavier, which can cause worry, but this is usually because you have left the hospital where you were resting and lying down and have now increased your activity, which triggers a heavier flow. This is another means Mother Nature uses to tell mums to slow down after giving birth. So don't try to do too much, too soon!

Your blood will go through different colour stages, from bright pink to a brownish colour and then finally a white discharge before it ceases. This process can take anywhere from a couple of weeks to six weeks. It is all part of the uterus healing and returning to its pre-pregnancy size, which I personally think is an incredibly short time considering what your body has just done.

What's abnormal and when should I call my GP, midwife or public health nurse?

If you have a fever, the bleeding stays bright red after the first week and remains heavy and you'll need to check in with your doctor. The same goes for an unpleasant smell from the lochia or if you are in a lot of pain and discomfort. These are mild warning signs that you must heed.

However, there are other signs that indicate more serious problems. You must call an ambulance if:

- along with sudden heavy bleeding, you start to feel faint, dizzy and lightheaded;

- the blood clots are the size of a golf ball or bigger;

- your heartbeat starts to race;

- you experience palpitations;

- you become confused and restless.

It's likely you'll have a gut feeling if all is not well, but a handy rule of thumb regarding blood clots post-delivery is that if the clot is the size of a five-cent piece, that's Top okay; if the clots are bigger than a fifty-cent piece, tip that could be an indication of a problem. Trust your instincts, keep an eye on the blood flow and clot sizes and do not hesitate to ask for help if you feel it's needed.

Bleeding that's much heavier than normal lochia is called postpartum haemorrhage (PPH). Losing 500mls or more of blood within the first 24 hours is called primary postpartum haemorrhage; abnormal or heavy vaginal bleeding between 24 hours and 12 weeks is called secondary postpartum haemorrhage. There can be many reasons for this, the most common being that the uterus doesn't contract normally after you've delivered the placenta, possibly as a result of fragments of the placenta or the amniotic sac remaining in the uterus after birth, an infection, or both. About

1% of postpartum women have a late postpartum haemorrhage, so it's relatively rare, thankfully.

If you do suffer from PPH, you can be treated with antibiotics or you may need a minor operation to remove the rest of the placenta. In rare cases you might need a blood transfusion for a primary PPH, but this is rare. Once you are receiving the right treatment for postpartum haemorrhage, you should be fine. It will take time to recover from it, however, so again you need to rest, nourish yourself with good food and keep well hydrated to deal with the anaemia caused by the blood loss. Remember, ask for and accept all help that's offered to you at this time to aid and speed your recovery.[2]

Top tip

There are enough embarrassing aspects to birth and post-birth, so be proactive and try to anticipate potential problems. One good idea is to buy the bed mats that are used for toilet-training kids and use them post-pregnancy in case of accidents, so you don't run the risk of ruining and changing sheets!

Going home

This is where the fun really begins, but it's also the part you are least prepared for during your pregnancy. I remember packing my bag in the hospital and feeling a mixture of nerves and excitement. I was looking forward to being at home, but I was not looking forward to being on my own. I loved the comfort of hospital and the support of the nurses. I was also very nervous handling James, as he was so tiny.

---

2 If you'd like more information on this important topic, go to: https://www.rcog.org.uk/globalassets/documents/patients/patient-information-leaflets/pregnancy/pi-heavy-bleeding-after-birth-postpartum-haemorrhage.pdf.

This is really when your self-care needs to kick in, but it's often the first hurdle at which mums fall and start to neglect themselves. In the hospital you are being handed fluids, food and painkillers at regular intervals, so when you get home you need help, reminders and preparation to mind yourself. I had a feeding chart and a changing chart that I filled in for James, to keep me on track, and I found it really helpful. So why not have a special Mummy Chart just for you and your needs.

Don't let the Mummy Chart freak you out by thinking of it as an extra chore. I know you don't have much time for lists and double-checking, so just put a tick beside the time you have eaten, had some fluids or managed to rest. It just gives you some idea of how your day is going and reminds you to do right by yourself, too.

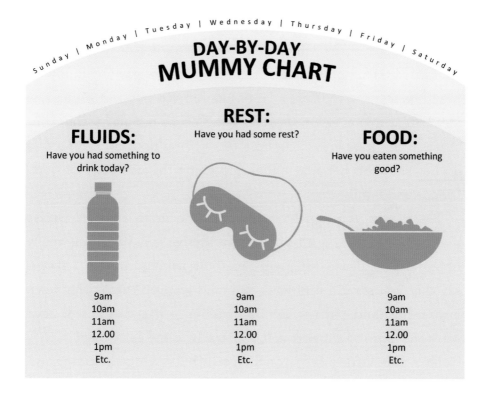

Sunday | Monday | Tuesday | Wednesday | Thursday | Friday | Saturday

DAY-BY-DAY
MUMMY CHART

REST:
Have you had some rest?

FLUIDS:
Have you had something to drink today?

FOOD:
Have you eaten something good?

FLUIDS	REST	FOOD
9am	9am	9am
10am	10am	10am
11am	11am	11am
12.00	12.00	12.00
1pm	1pm	1pm
Etc.	Etc.	Etc.

Keep this chart somewhere visible, like on the fridge or on the wall beside your baby's changing station, and set a couple of alarms throughout the day on your phone reminding you to mind yourself. Simply put into the alarm the message: ME. This might sound simplistic, but it's very easy to go the whole day when you have a newborn and not think about yourself at all. It's easy to leave long gaps between meals and get caught up in housework and washing when the baby is asleep. If visitors are coming, let them make you tea and not the other way around. If a partner, grandparent or friend offers to mind the baby for an hour while you nap, forget the housework and hit the sack. You can download a feeding chart from www.alisoncanavan.com.

Before you even go into hospital, batch-cook and freeze meals so that when you come out you don't have to worry about cooking. Your partner, husband or family member can continue this during the first few months, which will help ease a lot of pressure and stress. This is simply one less thing for you to worry about. If your friends want to visit, have a HSM lunch: Help Support Mum. The idea here is that everyone is given a job. Some people set the table, others bring food and clean up after, leaving nothing for mum to do but show off her new angel and enjoy the company of good friends and family.

The longer your newborn is home, the more you will realise that babies require a lot of work. In the early days help is really important, so please don't feel bad about asking for help. I always say that you should find your rock and lean on them, whether it is your husband, partner, family member or friend. You will need someone close to support you, especially in the early days.

Most parents do just fine on their own, but having a helping hand, or indeed hiring a helping hand if you can afford it, will make the adjustment into parenthood that bit easier. A relative could come and stay, for example, or there is a wide range of services on offer these days to cater for pretty much anyone's needs. There are day nurses, night nurses, nannies, au pairs or even a local babysitter to watch your other children for a couple of hours a day. Think about it before the birth and have a few action plans up your sleeve to help you recover and transition into your new family group.

Having help and support does not make you a bad mum. It does not mean that you can't cope with your responsibilities on your own, which I naively thought when I had James. I felt I had to do everything because I presumed other mums did, but getting help simply gives you the time to concentrate on your baby's needs and not on entertaining guests, making tea, cooking dinners and doing washing. The house will not fall down, and so what if it gets untidy during those early days? It will prepare you for the chaos of toddler times!

Top tip

Listen to your own instincts – if you need extra time to rest or be on your own, tell the people around you and let them help you to pencil in that time. Ask for help and don't beat yourself up about it – it's just an interim measure to get you fully back on your feet. If you are feeling a bit crowded by visitors, tell people you need some space and don't feel guilty about doing so. Friends with babies will understand. And if anyone doesn't understand, well, they aren't what matters right now – your feelings and wellbeing are the primary concern.

Relax and enjoy it!

The early days with your new baby can be full of stress and worry, which benefits no one. As the quote from Leo Buscaglia says: *Worry never robs tomorrow of its sorrow, it only saps today of its joy.* This is incredibly important to remember, especially in the early days when you are coming to terms with so many different things. There are so many things we worry about in our lives – our jobs, money, friends, family, illness – but worrying just stops you enjoying what is happening right now. My mind used to race all the time about tomorrow, work, getting organised and trying to find time in between feeds to get more stuff done. In the end, I realised that this stuff is usually unnecessary and can wait. Start catching these thoughts and try to question and rationalise them. Ask yourself if what you are doing really needs to be done or if it can wait. Could you perhaps take a 10-minute nap or even just sit on the couch instead of running to the grocery store? Be realistic about what you can do in a day, take it easy and, again, ask for help.

In the early days you will worry about feeding your baby, changing your baby, how much sleep your baby is getting and, if you are anything like me, you will obsessively check that they are breathing. I even woke James up once after a long night to make sure he was breathing and my own Mum nearly killed me because I was so tired! You see, we all do these things and they are completely normal, but I promise you that as time passes you will become comfortable with all of them. In the midst of all this, just make sure you don't forget about yourself along the way. Have you been changed, washed and fed? You might laugh at this or think it sounds silly, but you would be surprised at the amount of mums who do forget. There were many days my body never saw daytime clothes and even though that's okay once in a while, if it becomes a habit it can be bad for your emotional wellbeing.

You will hear people say to you over and over to enjoy your baby because they grow so fast. People used to drive me crazy saying it and the fact that we hear it so much is probably the reason most of us take no notice. But it's the old cliché of the truth being in the cliché: it is by far the most important thing you will be told. We unintentionally wish away almost every stage in our babies' lives. From the moment our babies are born we are trying to advance them to the next stage. We prop them up with cushions to sit, and then we force them to hold objects when they are not ready and then we help them stand and walk by holding their arms up. We ignore all these wise people who tell us to relax and enjoy them now as it will go by so fast.

When James was just a few weeks old, being pregnant felt like a distant memory and I was feeling lonely and vulnerable in my new role as a mum. I was also one of the first in my group of friends to have a baby. If you are feeling like this and it's affecting your ability to enjoy your baby, it is a good idea to join a local mum and baby group. Your local healthcare centre will have information or you can look online for a local class. I was really nervous attending my first mum and baby group, but you just need to remember that everyone is in the same boat. The people who run them are well aware of how nervous mums can be, especially if you are a first-time mum. Believe me, they will look after you when you arrive.

On difficult days, online forums can be useful and supportive. One of my friends became part of a Facebook page called March Mums – everyone on the page had babies born in March the same year. These informal communities are very helpful and can offer great support in the early days. Through them, you will find out you are all going through similar emotional and adjustment issues and that can be a comfort in itself. One word of caution: just be careful not to compare yourself with other mums because we are all different and how we cope, our body size, our sleep and indeed our babies will vary hugely. This might sound like I'm contradicting myself, but seeking support is very different from comparing yourself with other mums, which does nothing but make you feel inadequate and insecure.

Confidence can be an issue post-birth for so many reasons (I will discuss this in more detail in Chapter 4), but trusting yourself is the key. In the early days you will question your instincts, but if you relax, have some 'me time' and try to reduce stress, you will find that you will be in a better position to tune in and listen to yourself.

You have just come through the greatest physical event of your life and you are now facing the transition to a completely new life. It's a huge change and shouldn't be underestimated. It can be difficult, but time always softens the sharp edges of change and smoothens it out. You can help yourself by embracing the transition: don't mourn the past that's gone, look to the future with relish. This is a brand new beginning, with fresh hopes and dreams for both yourself, your child and your family. Sometimes we resist change and we can be scared of it and that's understandable, but if you embrace change, you embrace all the new adventures that life has to offer you. This is the most magical, rewarding, frustrating and exhausting journey you will ever embark on, but overall I believe it is the best thing you will ever do in your life. So from one mum to another, enjoy your journey.

What to expect in the early days

We have covered a lot of ground in this chapter and if you're soon to become a first-time mum, it's probably all a bit head-spinning. So let's look over the key points of what it will be like in the days and weeks after giving birth.

You are human and complicated and emotional: you will experience a wide range of emotions within a week and it's okay. Don't beat yourself up for 'negative' feelings – just be honest with yourself about each new feeling and know that it will pass. Things will keep changing and moving on.

You could be exhausted, or elated, or both: we are all different and your experience of your new baby will be unique. Don't bother comparing yourself to friends or family members. Listen politely if they insist on telling you how they fit into their size 8 jeans two days after giving birth, then let it go. It's nothing to do with you and your baby and your experience. Your only concern is you and how you feel.

You will experience varying degrees of pain post-birth: again, your experience is unique and will depend on your birth experience and what happened in the delivery room. Don't listen to anyone who wants to marvel at how different their experience was from yours.

It will take a while to feel comfortable in your body again: this is completely normal and you need to ease up on the demands you place on yourself. For a first baby, you can expect to need about 18 months before you feel like your pre-pregnant self; for each subsequent baby, it takes about two years.

It's quite likely you feel stress and worry: this is okay, you've had a major life event and you are trying to adjust to it. But try to take onboard the advice in this book and put in place whatever de-stressing techniques work for you. They are essential for your wellbeing, so put it on your To Do list along with all the baby shopping.

You might feel scared and vulnerable: there's a common idea that post-birth we are loved-up and happy, but this is not always the case. If your feelings are troubling you, surround yourself with people you love and who make you feel safe.

This is your early days survival guide!

* Trust yourself and listen to your instincts.

* Remember that food is your friend and don't forget to eat – especially if you are breastfeeding.

* Hydration is key: fluids, fluids, fluids.

* Get out for short walks – it will help clear your head and the fresh air is great for you.

* Speak up and ask questions of the professionals who are there to help you.

* Ask for help when you need it; accept help when it's offered.

* Sleep when the baby sleeps.

* Mum's only duties should be feeding and caring for herself and baby.

* Join a local mum and baby group.

* Be kind to yourself, your body and your emotions.

* If you are struggling with breastfeeding, seek support from a local group or lactation consultant.

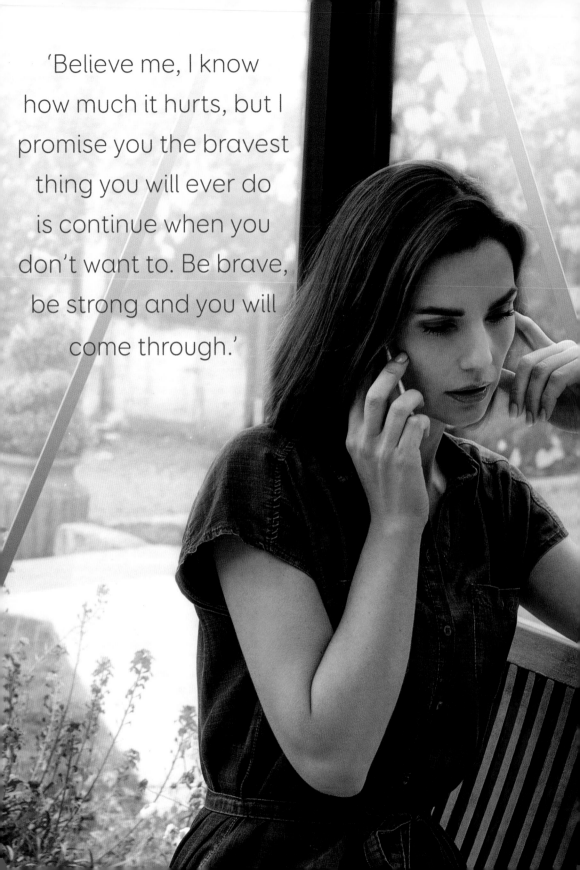

'Believe me, I know how much it hurts, but I promise you the bravest thing you will ever do is continue when you don't want to. Be brave, be strong and you will come through.'

3

BABY BLUES AND POST-NATAL DEPRESSION (PND)

This is by far the most difficult chapter for me to write because it reflects one of the most difficult times of my life, but it is also the most important chapter in this book for so many reasons. Even if you have never suffered any kind of mental health issues, I would love you to read this chapter because information is power and after a baby your life can be turned upside-down. This chapter will explain all about the baby blues and post-natal depression (PND) so that you can not only see warning signals for yourself but also for other mums. As mums we need to support each other and watch out for each other. Mums work great as a team, so choose teamwork every time rather than going it alone, it just makes sense.

It's a beautiful sunny day here today and this morning James and I went to the park. We stayed for two hours and he kept saying, 'Mum, stop kissing me and hugging me so much' and in the car he asked me if I was okay. He's not yet five years of age, but kids are incredibly perceptive. I'm an annoyingly positive mum, one who insists the first thing we do when we wake up in the morning is to say *Thank you for today*. Then we stretch and both go and drink some water. Some days we do yoga together and James watches me meditate most days, too. James is most certainly not used to seeing me sad because I believe in living a positive life; on bad days, I just try harder. I have had many bad days in my lifetime but luckily, because of how I have overhauled my lifestyle in the last few years, more recently I have had pretty much none at all.

The truth is, this is the fifth time I have sat down to write this chapter so this morning, at the park, I probably was apprehensive and didn't even realise it. I thought about hiding out in the playground for the whole day, but I knew I had to get home and just sit down and work through it. When you are in a good place it's very hard to dig up old feelings and hurtful memories. When James asked me why I was sad, I told him I was writing a book because sometimes mums get sad and this book will hopefully help new mums who are sad to feel happy again. He said that, luckily, I was an old mum now so I wouldn't be sad again. (I told him I was 21, he said 31 – so I gave in and admitted to that, even though I'm really 37!) He then told me that it was a great idea because no one should feel sad and he knows because he feels that way when he can't have sweets! So I have a five-year-old's blessing for this chapter, sprinkled with a touch of candy bribery. Here we go.

The passing of time can make a difficult period in your life not seem quite as bad as you once thought. I had been living with my Mum for a while after I had James and recently Mum had sold the family home. When she was moving out and I was helping with the packing up, I found a diary in my old room that I had kept from the day I discovered I was expecting a baby.

Why did I keep this diary? Well, I asked myself the same question. Journaling is a great way to help you cope with emotions and for me it's a form of therapy. When I discovered I was expecting I was newly single, in my early thirties and back living with my Mum. After living on Central Park West in NYC, it's safe to say it was all a bit of a shock. I was trying to cope with the fact that life can change in a split-second and for me it was that second when I found out I was pregnant. I knew that from then on my life would never be the same again.

Somewhat nervous, I sat on the couch in front of the fire in my new cosy comfortable little cottage and I began to read back on a journey that I had either chosen to forget or blocked out completely. Not all of it was bad, though. There were certainly lots of very happy parts and I cried at both in equal measure.

Just a few days after I had read my diary I received an e-mail from a mum who was suffering from post-natal depression and whose emotions were still very raw. Her words jumped off the page and straight into my heart and I felt her pain exactly like it was my own. I wondered about my own recovery and how much of it was masked in denial. It's so important to be true to ourselves in this life, especially if we want to be healthy and happy. To that end, I'll share my tips for recovery with you a little later on.

I felt that reading my diary was part two of my recovery – the part I wasn't strong enough to deal with first time round. Writing this book is the final stage and truly a dream come true for me. It has been said that we never get an opportunity to thank our real heroes in life and so now I would like to thank the hundreds of mums who took the time to write to me after I told my story on *The Late Late Show* and on various radio shows. I was so incredibly nervous when I spoke out publicly about my post-natal depression. But then, on some of the toughest days you can imagine, when I would genuinely feel like giving up, I would open my e-mails just at the right time to read a beautiful letter from a mum written straight from the heart. Those letters helped me hugely, and to each and every one of those mums I am deeply and truly grateful. You said in your e-mails and messages that I inspired you but really, you inspired me. It was as if the universe sent you as angels just at the right moment.

There were definitely diary entries earlier on that suggested I was beginning to struggle, like this one:

> 23 September 2010 (seven days after James was born)
> I need to rest more. I'm not superwoman. I'm starting to get tired and I need to watch my moods but I'm eating very well and really healthy so that's a plus.

It's important to note that these are normal feelings and emotions for any new mum, especially a week after giving birth. It's when these feelings persist and get worse over time that you need to think about asking for help.

There was one major warning sign I noticed in my diary, written on Wednesday, 20 October:

> I feel like I'm having a nervous breakdown at the moment and my world is crumbling. Let's hope I feel better tomorrow.

This was probably the moment when I needed to ask for help or tell someone I was struggling, but I didn't. I hid it and I just kept going and pushed and pushed myself until eventually I had no more to give.

To be honest, I don't remember writing the final part of my diary and not one word was written after this, but it is there in black and white. Today, I don't recognise the person who wrote it, but I'm really proud of her. The reason I'm sharing this is that I'm here today and doing better than ever. My son is my life and I'm finally incredibly happy and healthy and if there's even one mum out there that this helps, well then it's all been worthwhile. If any mum out there feels worried that she will never be herself again, I'm here to tell you that you can be and you will be. You need to mind yourself and take baby steps every day to get back on track, but you will get there.

The final diary entries, before I sought help:

14 February 2011
Besides crappy Valentine's Day I feel shit and James is sick. I hate feeling like this. I feel like a caged animal that can't escape. It's a mixture of anger, self-hatred and frustration. I hate my sisters but love them at the same time. I don't want pity or anything of the sort. I genuinely feel like falling down at any given time. Without James I would most certainly have had enough.

15 February 2011
Every day you push and stay positive and keep up your smile. I have no interest in anything right now. I feel guilty because of that. I feel like

such a burden. I can only imagine how they talk. I can't even support my own child. I wouldn't mind being in an accident and I think about wanting to die. That sentence lets me know I've hit rock bottom. The game's up. I've no more fight in me.

1 March 2011
My cousin makes me feel comfortable and safe and without her I don't know where I'd be. I feel trapped in myself, my voice unable to carry further than my mouth. I'm afraid of what people think. Why can't I cope? I hate people that pity themselves but a flicker of light at the end of the tunnel would be good.

I have a beautiful boy and he needs me. How many other mothers out there are feeling like this? I have asked for help but now I don't even want it. The thought of having to explain myself is gruelling and I'm tired just thinking about it.

Reading these words back was one of the most difficult things I have ever done in this lifetime. We live in a funny make-believe world sometimes, but a little bit of honesty goes a long way and I really wish I had known that most mums shed a few tears after having a baby and that the fact that I was finding it difficult to cope, especially in the early days, did not make me a bad mum, it made me a normal mum. Now I can look back and see that these words were the end of a nightmare and the beginning of the rest of my life because it was just after this that I sought help. I worked hard on myself from the inside out and today I am the healthiest I have ever been.

There is no denying that having a baby is a very special time in a woman's life. You want everything to be perfect and we all want to be great parents. We attend ante-natal classes, read books and devour every bit of information about pregnancy and birth. But what about after the baby is born? Research shows that at least 60% of women will struggle significantly during the first six months. That's a very high percentage for a subject that's simply not discussed. I had a great pregnancy after the sickness subsided at five months! I was so excited and couldn't wait to meet my baby. The birth was amazing and it's very empowering as a woman to bring a new life into the world. In the days that followed I grew to love James in a way I'd never felt before, an unconditional love that can only exist between a mother and her child.

The next few weeks were tough, but I still felt good. I seemed to be on top of everything and positive about my abilities as a new mum. But as I'm self-employed, I had to return to work quickly and I had some emotional problems going on as well. I was lucky to be able to bring James to work with me most of the time and my agent, Rebecca Morgan, let me bring him into the office every day. (Her patience and understanding is something I will never forget and I love her dearly.) But the lack of sleep was beginning to take its toll on me and I found myself crying for no apparent reason. The simple things became difficult and I felt like the world was caving in. Here I was with this beautiful little boy who was everything to me, but all I kept doing was bursting into tears. I couldn't understand it. James was a very good baby and I had my Mum around, who was also a great help. I felt like such a bad Mum.

> **I promise you that taking steps towards making yourself better is the greatest gift you will ever give yourself and your family.**

I also felt angry, ungrateful and ashamed. I'm a strong character and, to be honest, I was embarrassed to admit that I was having problems. I was also a person who adored babies and I've been looking after babies all my life. I couldn't understand how I could be so good with other people's babies but not with my own. It was this type of thinking that plunged me into a deeper depression.

I went from crying all the time to being completely unable to cope with the simplest of tasks. Daily life was completely overwhelming and I remember suffering a chronic panic/anxiety attack in a shopping centre one day. I was overwhelmed and couldn't cope, but I was ashamed to ask for help because I thought everyone would judge me. I also found it difficult to sleep, as I was so worried about everything. I avoided taking naps because as soon as I lay down I would start to think, which led me to worry. I had suffered from depression in the past and I recognised some signs. That was when I started to read up on the baby blues and post-natal depression. I was a textbook case. My mornings were becoming increasingly difficult. I felt so low that I didn't want to talk to friends or see anyone. I knew this was wrong. Finally, with the support of my family, I asked for help. I rang PND Ireland and a lady called Madge Fogarty spent an enormous amount of time on the phone with me; I will always be very grateful to her for her time and help.

I began counselling and went to a psychiatrist and took medication. I took baby steps and began to educate myself even more about food and lifestyle. Medication has its place for some people and it can definitely be a step on the ladder to recovery, but

I just knew, deep down, that there had to be more to all this than taking pills. I was sick of popping pills to fix my problems. I cleaned up my lifestyle and began to understand the power of living better, which was a lifestyle I had always regarded as boring. In fact, I learned pretty quickly that it's not boring at all – it's amazing!

During my recovery I began to research human happiness and although everyone has a different opinion on this subject, they are all very interesting and thought-provoking. One thing is for sure, though: it definitely comes from within.

> "Most of us have no idea what it actually feels like to be happy naturally and that's a shame."

From a personal perspective, I think we have all grown up in a world that is simply moving far too fast for us and many of us are struggling to keep up most of the time. From an early age we are eating processed food and a lot of teenagers give up physical exercise in their late teens. That's also when many people start experimenting with alcohol and drugs. As a result, our ability to feel good naturally is taken away from us at a young age. As we get older, we begin to rely on stimulants or multiple outside sources for happiness.

When people decide they want to live a healthier life, feel better and lose weight, they often try to overhaul all of their bad habits in one go. What most don't realise is that everyone will go through some form of healing crisis and feel worse before they feel better. I believe this is the reason why most people fail when they try to change their ways; they don't push past that point to get to the other side.

Facing my depression and anxiety was incredibly painful and I felt like throwing in the towel many times but I also desperately wanted to get better, so I persevered, sometimes just with the mere hope that I would come out the other end. Eventually I did, and my diagnosis of

Pyroluria definitely helped, but I also genuinely believe that with the correct support and help everyone can recover and that our lifestyle choices play a big part in this too. You just need to understand the journey: it's not going to be easy, but it will be worth it.

Post-natal depression doesn't discriminate, it can affect any mum regardless of situation or age. You can suffer on your first or your fourth child, which is important to remember because if you didn't suffer on previous children, you can be very hard on yourself if you do become ill.

Being a first-time mum is really daunting. You're handed your little bundle and sent on your way. It's a time of huge adjustment and responsibility. Throw into the mix a few hormones and lack of sleep and your world very simply gets turned upside-down. There's an enormous pressure to be a 'supermum' nowadays. It's a perfect storm of negative associations, capable of eclipsing your self-esteem and self-trust. My advice for coping is very simple: go easy on yourself and trust your instincts.

A closer look at the baby blues and PND

Before we begin I would like to mention that there is such a thing as ante-natal depression, which is referred to as pre-natal depression.

Pre-natal depression can present with symptoms such as:

* anxiety;

* sleep problems;

- feeling irritable in yourself and with those around you;

- harbouring fears about the future;

- appetite loss;

- tired all the time – you might even want to stay in bed;

- becoming withdrawn.

Pregnancy is an emotional time and your hormones are rampaging freely throughout your body and could be causing a bit of trouble. Your pregnancy might be unplanned, uncomfortable or complicated. The bottom line is that there are many reasons you might start to feel down, but the important thing is that you ask for help because pre-natal depression can be a precursor to post-natal depression if not properly treated. It is estimated that 7–20% of pregnant women are affected by this condition.[3]

According to Dr Edmond O'Flaherty: 'During pregnancy copper is an essential element in the body (responsible for over 20 reactions) and during pregnancy it's involved in making blood vessels for the baby. In the third trimester copper doubles (and maybe a bit higher!) and if the copper level doesn't drop off after you give birth, PND is likely. In some women it can take months before it settles down. Because of higher copper levels it is thought that PND can even start before birth. You can bring it down naturally with zinc – typically 50mg a day after delivery.'

---

3 See http://journals.lww.com/greenjournal/Abstract/2004/04000/Prevalence_of_Depression_During_Pregnancy_.16.aspx and https://www.health.ny.gov/community/pregnancy/health_care/perinatal/perinatal_depression.htm.

Baby blues

After birth your body changes dramatically and between your hormone levels, your sore breasts and being tired, is it any wonder you feel a little blue? In fact, if you don't feel like crying in the weeks after your baby is born, then you are one of the very lucky ones because various studies have shown that between 60% and 70% of mums will experience the baby blues in some form. Some studies even state that up to 80% of mums suffer baby blues in some form. I would be leaning towards the 80% as I have yet to meet a mum who didn't struggle even a little bit.

What are the symptoms of the baby blues?

The main symptoms are very simple:

* crying;

* feeling really sad.

If you find yourself bursting into tears and feeling sad, don't panic – you are most certainly not alone. It's important to know and understand that this is all completely normal and that these feelings usually disappear without help. A lot of women I have spoken to have said they remember just bursting into tears even though they weren't feeling sad. Sometimes tears are just a way of releasing emotions – if you haven't the energy or time to deal with them properly, they have to come out somehow.

If you are suffering from the baby blues you can also feel:

* fatigued;

* lonely;

* irritable;

* have difficulty sleeping; or

* have strong emotional reactions.

This is why it's really important to ask for and to accept help. I think I put pressure on myself to prove that I could cope because I already felt guilty about being a single mum. But your situation is irrelevant and here's why: baby blues, post-natal or any other kind of depression does not care if you are rich or poor, fat or thin, tall or small, old or young, married or unmarried, single or in a couple or anything else for that matter. Anyone can suffer at any time and for many different reasons. This is so important to understand because very often we judge with our eyes and depression is invisible. There is no one type of person who gets depression and it's really important that everyone understands this because no one knows what tomorrow holds or indeed what surprises life has in store for us.

> " Baby blues, post-natal or any other kind of depression does not care if you are rich or poor, fat or thin, tall or small, old or young, married or unmarried, single or in a couple or anything else for that matter. Anyone can suffer at any time and for many reasons. "

This is another reason why prevention and information are so important as they enable us to recognise the warning signs and to take necessary steps to help either ourselves, a friend or a family member.

What can you do to beat the blues?

* Good nourishing food.

* Talk to your friends, family and spouse/boyfriend and tell them how you feel. Ask for their help to get through this time.

* Try and get out for a walk. I know this is difficult for C-section mums in the early days, but do try and get some fresh air, otherwise you'll get severe cabin fever.

* Sleep when the baby sleeps (easy on your first, much harder if you have other children, but still equally important).

* Arm yourself with information. Helpful resources if you think you are suffering from post-natal depression include: **Post-Natal Depression Ireland**, Tel: 021-492 2083, www.pnd.ie; **Aware**, www.aware.ie; **Parentline**, Tel: 01 873 3500 or lo-call 1890 927 277, www.parentline.ie/info@parentline.ie.

When your blues become more serious

The baby blues should pass within a few days or at most a couple of weeks, but if you find you can't shake the feelings of sadness, you're crying all the time and have an inability to cope with day-to-day life, it's important to talk to someone and get the support you need. Post-natal depression can manifest itself in so many different ways and can be caused by so many different factors that it is very difficult to provide a definitive checklist for everyone, but health professionals use a method called the Edinburgh Scale to make assessments.

The Edinburgh Post-natal Depression Scale (EPDS) is a 10-item questionnaire that was developed to identify women with PND. (See www.alisoncanavan.com for the scale.) The questions focus on sleep, mood, guilty feelings, a lack of energy and suicidal thoughts.

The signs and symptoms of post-natal depression

Again, there is no definitive list as it will vary from individual to individual, but the common signs and symptoms are as follows:

* tiredness and/or an inability to sleep when given the opportunity;

* sleeping too much or too little;

* crying all the time;

* irritable;

* no interest in the things you usually enjoy;

* no interest in anything;

- depressed and low feelings;

- lack of motivation;

- anxiety and panic attacks;

- loss of appetite or comfort eating;

- a low sex drive;

- not enjoying the time with your baby and possibly even feeling hostile towards your baby;

- being completely overprotective of your baby and reluctant to let anyone help with him/her or hold him/her;

- being obsessed about your baby's health, watching them breathe constantly and taking them to the doctor all the time for the slightest little thing;

- a new baby can bring financial and emotional stress and if you're having relationship problems, this can also be a contributing factor;

- the simple everyday tasks seem overwhelming, like changing a nappy, dressing yourself or the baby, showering, making food, etc.;

- suicidal thoughts or thoughts about harming yourself and/or your baby;

- negative thoughts and feelings about yourself;

- no confidence;

- blaming yourself for everything;

- bonding issues with the baby – you might feel you don't love your baby enough;

- no interest in seeing anyone – friends or family.

(For comprehensive information on this topic, see www.hse.ie, which has a section on primary care for PND.)

While this list might not be exhaustive, there is one thing I can say for sure: early intervention is key. If the dark cloud does not lift, you have got to ask for help. The reality is that if you don't get help, it will get worse and you will deteriorate further. The good news is that early intervention or getting help as soon as you can means a faster recovery. Your baby needs you to be present. Forget about the housework and the washing and focus on you and your baby. Talk to someone close to you about how you're feeling. Recent research suggests that group therapy and talking about your feelings has a big part to play in recovering from depression. Since getting treatment, I now understand that it wasn't my fault.

If you have a public health nurse, talk to her or visit your GP and they can help you to take the next step. A good GP is essential as he/she will talk through your options and you can decide together the best route to recovery for you.

My advice is to contact a helpline, such as Parentline or PND Ireland (contact details on p.68). I found this to be a lifesaver in my own situation and I wouldn't hesitate to recommend Parentline or PND Ireland to others. It's a little easier to do because the person on the other end of the phone is fully trained, non-judgemental and they can't see you. So if you're struggling to take the first step towards tackling your negative feelings after birth, consider this option. It might just work for you, too.

My personal tips to help combat PND

* Try to get as much rest as possible. Sleep when the baby sleeps or ask someone to take the baby for a walk while you nap.

* Try to have at least a 10-minute walk every day with the baby.

* Taking small steps is the key, for example, take a shower. I know this can be hard when you're tired, but it will do wonders for how you're feeling.

* Keep a diary of how you feel and try to write down 10 positive things that happen each day no matter how small, even just 'changed a nappy' or 'fed the baby'. When you start to see what you are doing, you will stop focusing on what you're not doing.

* Eat well. A good breakfast is essential. Cut out fried, fatty and sugary foods. Food and nutrients are the most powerful medication we have.

* Join a local mum and baby group so you can ask questions and learn from other mums and it's also good to get out and about. Look online for listings in your area.

* Talk, talk, talk … tell someone if you're not feeling well or go online and talk to other mums and ask questions.

* Trust in yourself, 'Mum knows best', and know that you will return to the 'real you' soon.

* Talk to your GP about your options and, if necessary, find a good counsellor.

* As women we need to support each other more and try to be a bit more open and honest. If you feel your friend needs help, try to talk to her gently about how she's feeling.

Stop being so hard on yourself

As women we really do put a lot of pressure both on ourselves and on each other. We all parent differently and we are all individuals. If you really want to be the best, then be the best you that you can be because, as we all know, everyone else is taken.

Don't think for one second that you are the only person not coping or having tough days because we all are. That girl you see strolling through the park looking amazing a couple of weeks after having her baby might very simply be having a good day, or she might have spent the morning crying and put on that make-up to hide her pain. The thing is, we just don't know what goes on behind closed doors so don't compare and don't presume, instead be kind and supportive to yourself and others and if she looks great, see it as something to work towards for yourself and not something to envy or resent.

When I found it difficult to express myself verbally, I found that journaling really helped. It helped me to recognise certain feelings and understand them better. I have realised that I am incredibly hard on myself. For most of my life I have been so self-critical and, to be honest, I'm just exhausted by it all. I'm exhausted of being judged by people who don't know me and in turn, because of my lack of self-esteem and confidence, judging others. This is an unhealthy, unhelpful and very negative way to live. During my recovery from post-natal depression I learned that when I changed how I treated myself, my entire world and those in it also changed – for the better!

Dr Wayne Dyer, who is an internationally renowned author and speaker, put this beautifully: *'When you change the way you look at things, the things you look at change.'*

As you recover from post-natal depression, the good days will start to tip the scale in your favour. When that happens, you are on the home stretch. Now you just need to practice what I like to call mental maintenance.

Mental maintenance

Mental maintenance is something everyone should do to help prevent themselves from becoming ill with a 'Dis-Ease' of the mind. I like to use the term Dis-Ease because I truly believe that mental health is just like any other illness, in other words when we are unwell it's because an element of us, either mentally or physically, is at Dis-Ease.

"

One only sees what one looks for, one only looks for what one knows.

Goethe

"

Through my struggle and recovery from depression and anxiety I have learned the power of self-care, resilience, emotional and physical wellbeing and so much more. It took 20 years for me to have that *Aha!* moment when I realised that nothing works in isolation and that our body, mind and spirit are one, which means that if one is out of balance, it will knock the others off too. We need to find our own formula and balance our own scales. I say 'our own' because we are all different and what works for one person will not work for another. Just because your friend saw a certain therapist, took a certain exercise class, took a certain medication and said it worked for them, it does not necessarily follow that it will work for you.

Get out there and figure out what makes you happy. You need to nurture yourself from the inside out in order to take care of your mind. Eat great food, get outside, and talk kindly to and about yourself and others. Find your passion and follow it and start each day with gratitude for simply being here.

Our mental health is something that is not visible to the human eye and because of that we find it very difficult to comprehend and cope with. Very often we will ignore it, hoping our problems will go away and tomorrow will be a better day, but unfortunately most of the time this is not the case.

Our society tends to stick plasters on problems as they arise, but it's important to know that there is an awful lot we can do to prevent having to use plasters at all. Most of us think that these things will never happen to us, but no one knows what life has in store. My experience with my own mental health has humbled me and I see so much beauty now in a world that seemed so harsh and cruel before. I am so grateful for my health and I practice mental maintenance every day. Even though it can be hard staying well, it's definitely far easier than getting sick and starting all over again.

What I most want you to take from this discussion

The one thing I would love to help achieve is the removal of any and all stigma surrounding depression. We can't see depression and I really do understand how difficult it must be to comprehend for someone who has never experienced it. As a result, it is a silent killer. That's why I was terrified to tell anyone how I was feeling for so long and even when I was sick and spoke out, people often commented that I didn't look unwell. For years I was terrified of being judged, so I suffered in silence, caught in a cycle of self-medicating and feeling angry with myself for feeling the way that I did.

Depression is not like a broken arm or a cut or a bruise, something tangible and easy to treat, but the pain it causes is very real. I often think that if we could see depression, if it took a form, we would be unable to look for long as it would be too hard. We all need to open our hearts, to open our minds and try to see beyond our own mind's limitations. The more mental health is accepted and talked about, the more people will get help sooner and also those around them will have the confidence and courage to speak up. Life is a team sport and you have to be in to win. So whether you are a support to someone with a brain Dis-Ease or a sufferer of a Dis-Ease within your own brain, you need to recognise it, accept it and then take steps to deal with it.

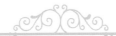

The key to solving the problem:
talk – ask – do.

Talk to someone and let him/her know there's a problem (this could also be a helpline, as suggested above), or be there for someone who wants to talk to you.
Ask for help and get referred to someone who can help you.
Do whatever it takes to get well, or do whatever it takes to help someone get well.

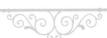

> **"** *Don't suffer in silence* **"** From my own experience I learned that you must own your feelings and acknowledge them and then try to work through them. You can't just wake up and expect this to go away, but with the right support and help you will recover, and quicker than you think. I took baby steps and lived day by day, which helped me to focus on the present and appreciate what I had. Worrying about the future does nothing but cause anxiety.

So to all the mums out there in pain, please:

* don't suffer in silence;

* early intervention means you will get better quickly;

* believe you will get better;

* believe in yourself.

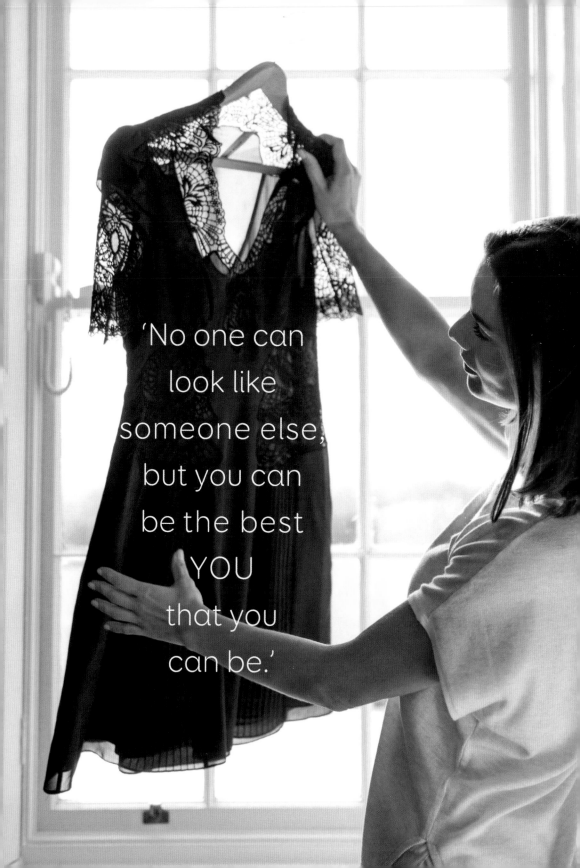

'No one can
look like
someone else,
but you can
be the best
YOU
that you
can be.'

YOUR POST-BABY BODY AND BODY IMAGE

4

I have to be honest, after I gave birth I felt like an imposter in my new body, waiting for my old body to return. I naively thought that as I was a model and had never had any weight issues, my body would pop back into shape post-birth. My Mum had five kids and always seemed to shed any baby weight pretty easily, so I should have nothing to worry about, right?

Wrong! The body I had handed over for nine months as a baby-making machine was now pulled out of shape and I felt a bit like playdough that needed to be moulded back to its original form. I had stretchmarks and cellulite where there was previously none. It can be hard to accept, but just remember that your new body has created a miracle, given birth to a miracle and, believe it or not, left behind a miracle and that miracle is you. You need to respect the miracle in all its glory, big, small, stretchy, not so stretchy anymore and give yourself a break!

Just think about what our little miracle machines do:

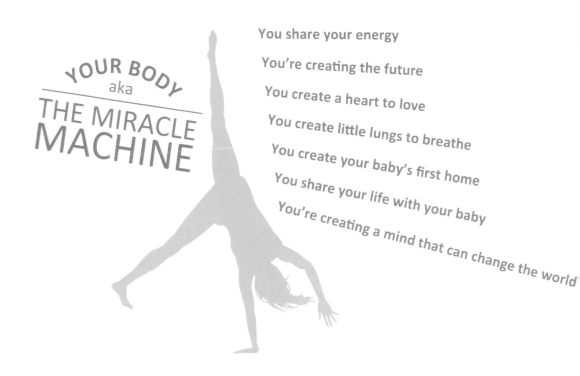

YOUR BODY aka THE MIRACLE MACHINE

You share your energy

You're creating the future

You create a heart to love

You create little lungs to breathe

You create your baby's first home

You share your life with your baby

You're creating a mind that can change the world

I lost the initial baby weight quite quickly, but I really struggled with the last 10 lbs or so. We are all different and we will all have different stories, but one thing remains the same: we all need to be kind to ourselves. After I gave birth it was the first time in my life I really cursed my career choice because as a single mother my income depended on my body size (not on my feelings) and with no maternity pay, I had to get back to clothes-horse size pretty quickly. I use the term clothes-horse here because during this time I really began to realise how ridiculous my job can be sometimes and how much pressure I place on myself. But please listen because I was the crazy new mum who did crazy things so you don't have to.

I also suffered from post-natal depression, as I've described in Chapter 3, and during this time I comfort ate. I kept a diary during my pregnancy and after, and here is one entry that shows how mean we can be to ourselves:

> I got some new clothes today that actually fit me as I feel like a fat cow and I have put on so much weight. I really need to stop and control my eating. That probably means dealing with why I'm eating first.

The next day I wrote:

> I tried on all my jeans today and nothing fits so I went shopping and tried on jeans that I thought were a size 12 and they fit but they were an American size 12, which is a UK 16. I nearly had a heart attack. I need to lose weight quick to work but I feel sad and eating makes me feel better.

This might seem like an extreme reaction, but this is honestly what was going through my head at the time and I'm sure it's very common. Writing this today I am certainly quite horrified by how I spoke to myself and what I thought of myself back then, but it really proves that our individual problems are our own and they are huge to us. Remember, I had been influenced by a world of unreality.

What I have learned is that no one's body is the same and no one can look exactly like someone else, but we need to be happy in our own skin and the only way we can achieve this is by living healthily and eating well. By doing these simple things you can be the best you. Living healthily will also increase your confidence (so you won't say awful things to yourself, like I did) and help you to feel better all over.

I am naturally thin and never really had to work at it for the first 12 to 15 years of my career, but I have lived through incredibly insecure times since giving birth and now I understand what it's like to struggle to lose weight. Throughout my career when work dipped and I felt sad, I used all sorts of escapisms, including over-eating, alcohol, diet pills, no food and excessive exercise. The sad truth is: I was completely miserable throughout these times.

Learning to love my post-baby body was the first time I had ever consciously loved my body. I now respect my body, which was something I certainly never did before. I thought about how much I cherished and nurtured my body with a baby growing inside it and wondered why I didn't feel that way all the time, especially when the baby came out. The fact that I would always put someone else first, especially my baby, was very telling about the nature and journey of motherhood. Just look at how any animal protects its young – there is simply nothing you wouldn't risk or do to protect your newborn, even when it's inside you. It's natural to protect both your unborn child and your newborn, but we have to make the space to protect and mind ourselves too. If you don't create that space for yourself, you'll become exhausted and resentful and those feelings will threaten your family's happiness. It benefits everyone when you take a sensible approach to parenting and 'me time'.

It took time and a lot of cake and tears, but I have now learned to love and respect my new body. It was difficult, but I think it's probably difficult for every woman. It's all too easy to wear the slouchy clothes, eat the sugary foods and tell yourself it's for the good of your baby. That will be fine for a few weeks, but inevitably it will catch up on you and you'll find yourself with low energy, up-and-down hormones, bad skin and weight gain. Those things will in turn make you feel awful about yourself, and you might well try to drown those bad thoughts in ice cream, chocolate or wine. It's a truly vicious circle. The good news is, you have the power to smash through that circle right now and change how you feel. So I'm giving you permission to congratulate your body and give it some R&R, feel free to take it for naps, rub cream on it, wear comfy clothes and you can even take it out for a few hours or on a day trip to a spa for some treatments. Why? Because you deserve it!

> " *We all need to learn to love the body we are in as it's the only one we have.* "

I often hear mums say (and indeed I said it myself), 'I wish I had my pre-baby body back', but can you honestly tell me you didn't moan about your pre-baby body, too? Once you have given your body time to really heal and recover, then you can begin getting used to your new body and learn to accept it. In the meantime, dressing our 'inbetweener' body is definitely a challenge, so here are some tips that might help.

Dressing your post-baby body

Without a doubt, one of my finest 'model moments' was when I packed my pre-pregnancy clothes into my hospital bag without a second thought. I actually brought them to the hospital, if you can believe that. Of course, I soon realised that, much to my disappointment, I wasn't Superwoman and I asked my Mum to bring in my wine-coloured maternity dress as it was far more comfortable! I most certainly did not admit what I had just done to Mum; I just had a quiet giggle about it.

In the days and weeks after I gave birth, I noticed that my actual body shape had changed quite considerably. Even after I had regained my figure, my old clothes just didn't fit right – after all, our hips do move during pregnancy and childbirth! I also found that my weight was distributed differently so my old dresses and jeans were simply not comfortable anymore.

I had to learn how to dress post-birth, and then I had to learn that pregnancy is a point of no return – you can't go back to before, so you have to accept how you are in the present.

So there are a couple of things you need to be aware of and think about:

* dressing your body as it changes in the weeks and months post-birth;

* getting to know and love your new body.

Dressing your body as it changes in the weeks and months post-birth

It takes at least six to eight weeks for your uterus to contract post-birth, so needless to say some of your pregnancy clothes can become your post-pregnancy clothes for a while. Immediately post-pregnancy my number one rule is: Comfort is Key.

Believe it or not, you can be comfortable, stylish, feel good and look well after a baby. I'm well aware you are exhausted and that sentence might only make you feel even more tired, but stay with me. Here are some helpful ways to look good post-birth without too much hassle.

* **Use shapewear or a bellyband** (www.bellybandit.com). I used shapewear all the time after the baby was born. It can be very helpful to have an extra layer of fabric holding you in and there's a feeling of comfort and confidence when you are being held in, too. (I didn't have a C-section, but some of my friends who did said that wearing bellybands helped make them feel more supported and comfortable.) Bellybands and belly belt-extenders are great. Most maternity stores stock a variety of these and you can even buy combo kits online. They allow you to wear your regular jeans, trousers, shorts and skirts throughout pregnancy and afterwards. Waist-band extenders are also great for both button- and slide-fastening garments. They come in all different sizes and colours and, depending on your size, can enable you to get back into your pre-pregnancy jeans a lot quicker.

* I loved **Lycra tops designed for pregnancy** that grew with my bump and also shrunk with my belly, almost like comfy shapewear. I wore a fitted top under all my clothes as it helped me to feel more confident in myself.

* **Set aside some money to buy yourself some 'in-betweener' clothes.** This is where the high-street is your best friend. You do not have to spend much and this way you get to wear clothes that are in fashion and that fit, which will help you to feel good. I do have one rule about fashion, though, which I have stuck to throughout my career: wear what suits you and don't choose anything

just because it's on trend. Whatever is trending in fashion will not suit everyone, so for my part I choose elements of trends that work well for me. A good example of a trend that could work post-pregnancy is peplums on tops and dresses, which can help to hide a multitude. Invest in these clothes three to four weeks post-birth because most women will plateau then for a while and during this time you need to be resting and not exercising too much (or at all, except for walking – see Chapter 6).

Don't wear clothes that are too big or too small as both extremes are incredibly unflattering. Often we try to hide ourselves under baggy clothing, but in reality this just makes us look even bigger. The same applies when we try to squeeze ourselves into our pre-pregnancy clothes too soon – not attractive and very uncomfortable.

There are some **amazing maternity clothes** available that don't look like maternity clothes. By this I mean they have no ruching on the sides or a clear bump area. These are great to wear immediately post-birth and during your transitional period.

Make sure your trousers have Lycra in them and are stretchy for comfort and feel. This is particularly important if you have had a C-section. I would recommend yoga pants with a nice T-shirt for hanging out around the house (www.graceandaibell.com). As far as regular pants go, hipsters are out (you will be bending over a lot with a new baby). Find pants that fit you well and don't sit too low on the waist. Steer away from pants that are fancy and adorned with decorations and patterns or if they have huge pockets on the butt area, because these will just draw attention to the area and make you look bigger. If you wear fuller skirts or dresses that flare out a little or are A-line shaped, they will make you look more balanced from top to bottom and draw attention to your hips.

* **Wear your maternity jeans but turn the band down.** This worked well for me because it was comfortable and turning the band down secured the fit and draw attention from your hips.

* **A dressy silhouette can work wonders.** I just love dresses, they are simple and easy to wear and if you shop smart, you can find a shape to suit you perfectly. I wore my maternity dresses after birth and used belts of varying widths around my midriff, especially in the evenings or for special occasions. Thick, wide ribbons can be really beautiful too and will help you to hide any wobbly bits. You could also use embellished lace or velvet ribbons (especially if you are going somewhere dressy) in black, cream, deep red or teal green, for instance. These are a great way to glam up a simple dress, especially the old reliable LBD (little black dress). Pair the LBD with matching shoes and bag or matching jewellery for a comfortable but classy look.

* **If all else fails, go back to black.** Ah yes, you can't beat black on those days when nothing else will work.

Black makes bad days better and it can help to give you confidence, especially if you have an occasion like a wedding soon after having a baby. A trusted LBD can be dressed up or down. Black can be very elegant, slimming and sophisticated, so use it to your advantage.

* **Accessorise!** Jewellery can divert attention and take the eye away from your problem areas. The only drawback is that as your baby grows, their love for your jewellery will also grow, which can lead to a conflict of interests! However, there are some companies that sell beautiful jewellery that looks great and is safe for your baby to chew on – see, for example, www.mikabteethingjewellery.ie and www.crownchewels.co.uk.

> " *Black can help hide a multitude from sight, but bright and light will help put your mood right.* "

* **Add a pop of colour.** This is especially the case during the summer months when your wardrobe can start to reflect the brighter, fresher days. If you are somewhere warm, lighter, brighter fabrics and colours will also help to keep you cool. Adding a pop of colour to a rainy day can also do wonders for your mood. When I'm feeling down, I always make sure to wear a bright colour to lift my mood, even if it's just bright socks or a scarf.

* **Steer clear of loose pants and loose tops.** It balances your body shape better if you have fitted pants and a

loose top or the opposite, a fitted top and loose bottoms. The bottoms could be a skirt, jeans or trousers.

* **Stay in stretchy jeans until your uterus shrinks.** Stick to dark colours for jeans as they are more slimming and always remember that no one feels sexy in tracksuit bottoms. I know if I'm having a bad day, just getting dressed can make me feel better!

* **Use belts cleverly post-pregnancy.** They can be used over dresses but also over cardigans and long sweaters. Experiment with different looks and find the one that suits your shape best.

* **Glam it up!** A fabulous, colourful pair of shoes, a great bag, a nice silk ribbon to loosely tie a dress, a great hairdo, jewellery (even big statement earrings) and nice make-up will make you forget about your post-baby bump entirely! I would add a bright lip to this as well, if the night's right. Remember when you used to do this for fun as a child, playing dress-up? Well, you can still do it as an adult and have just as much fun!

* **Layer, layer, layer, especially in winter.** Dressing this way is something I had to learn to do when I lived in NYC to deal with the cold, but it's actually a far more practical way of dressing so you can take off layers. Bulky sweaters make you feel bigger, which is not what you need post-pregnancy, whereas thin layers help to make you feel slimmer.

Top tip

Wearing clothes that are either too tight or too loose is unflattering, uncomfortable and impractical for a busy mum. Get the right fit for you in everything you buy, then nothing will sit unworn in your wardrobe.

The Golden Rules, or what not to do when dressing your post-pregnancy body:

* don't wear what's in fashion, wear what suits your shape;

* don't try on your pre-pregnancy clothes for a while after having your baby – wait until you are pretty sure you have a chance of fitting into them, otherwise you'll commit confidence suicide;

* don't compare yourself to other women and celebs, which is also a surefire confidence killer;

* don't diet, instead eat energy-rich foods and thank your wonderful body for all the hard work;

* don't wear uncomfortable fabrics around your scar area if you have had a C-section. Choose cottons and stretchy pants.

Your breasts and your underwear

I have to admit, one of my favourite parts of being pregnant was a dramatically increased bra size. I was so happy to actually need a bra for the first time in my life that I invested in really nice underwear. I figured if they were going to be sore and leaky post-birth, I was at least going to dress them up. Some maternity bras can be ugly, but I'm a girl and let's be honest, nice things make you feel nice even if no one else can see them. Let me tell you, what you wear underneath your clothes can definitely impact on your confidence, just as much as what the world can see.

Having spent the majority of my youth stuffing bras and buying padded bras, I took great pride in asking the shop assistant for a bra with good support. Your bra size can change up to four times during your pregnancy and it's really important – especially if they are new, like mine were – that you get measured and fitted correctly throughout. My lovely full breasts are gone now, but it was nice while it lasted!

The experience of pregnancy is different for everyone and whether you experience a large or small increase in breast size one thing is for sure, regular fashion bras are not designed to provide the support and comfort you will need as your breasts grow heavier and become more sensitive.

A lot of women find wearing underwired bras uncomfortable and a lot of health professionals advise against them as they can interfere with the natural changes in the size and shape of your breasts and may obstruct the increased blood flow to your breasts during and post-pregnancy. Your breasts may become lumpy early on, as the milk duct system begins to develop, and if not fitted correctly underwired bras can press against your developing milk duct system and cause discomfort. Though there's no hard evidence that wearing them will cause any harm, I always err on the side of caution. If you do prefer a bra with wires, just make sure it is a specifically designed maternity bra with a wire support suitable for use during pregnancy and for breastfeeding.

Once you've outgrown your usual bras, you'll want a comfortable, non-wired maternity bra with soft but supportive cups. You can wear maternity bras in bed if your breasts need extra support when lying down. Some stores sell bras that have been specially designed for wearing in bed at night and I found these bras really comfortable and supportive for my new-found friends!

Maternity and nursing bras are designed to accommodate your enlarging breasts and expanding rib cage, are seamless and are made from soft, flexible material that makes them really comfortable to wear. They will also give you that extra support you need and when worn regularly can also help eliminate stretchmarks. I'm a huge fan of anything that might even have a slight chance of preventing stretchmarks!

You should buy your first maternity/nursing bras about four or five months into your pregnancy and you will need a minimum of three bras – one to wash, one to wear and one to have ready in case you have leaks during your time nursing. It's also important that they have one-handed access with lots of support and extendible clips, like BoobDesign Nursing Bra Fast Food. I love that title, Fast Food, as we all know that when a baby's hungry, fast food is essential, but at least this fast food is healthy.

Measuring for your bra

Most good maternity stores offer a free bra-fitting service and there are so many incredible companies around now selling great brands like Cache Coeur, Cake Lingerie, Belabumbum and BoobDesign (see, for example, www.cherishme.ie). They specialise in underwear designed for pregnancy and after, but also designed for women – pretty, sexy and fun.

First things first, though, you need to find your correct size. To do this, you will need to find out your cup size and your band size. Step A: the band measurement is the measurement taken around the body, just below the bust line. For your band measurement you will need to measure across the bottom of your band, directly under the bust and across your rib cage. Make sure to keep your measuring tape straight around the back to front. (Ask someone to help here, if necessary.) If you get an odd number, round it up to the next even number to get your band size.

Step B: to find your cup size, you need to get your bust measurement, which is the measurement taken around the body at the widest part of the bust. Measure loosely around the fullest part of your bust, with the tape straight across and around your back, bringing it to the front. Subtract your band measurement (Step A) from this bust measurement (Step B). The difference calculates your bra size and each inch represents a cup size.

The science part isn't always easy, so an example will help explain this.

If you measure a 37-inch bust size and a 34-inch band size, the difference is 3 inches, which makes you a 34C; or a 36-inch bust size and a 34-inch band, the difference here is 2 inches, which would indicate a B cup. If you'd prefer an expert to do it, stores like Mothercare and Marks & Spencer offer a great measuring and fitting service for pregnant and post-natal mums.

This chart explains it even more clearly:

The difference (in inches)	0	1	2	3	4	5	6	7
Your cup size is	AA	A	B	C	D	DD	DDD, F	G

Measuring can be done without a bra or when wearing a very light bra (with no padding). When taking the measurements, breathe out and try keeping the measuring tape level and horizontal with the floor. The good news is that most maternity bras have an adjustable back strap that allows you to adjust the bra size as your breast size changes throughout your pregnancy.

Do not be afraid to go up a cup size, if necessary. If you are measuring for your bra in your early pregnancy, it is good to keep in mind that your breasts will change throughout your pregnancy in both shape and size and that you may also need to leave space for breast pads, if nursing.

When measuring for your bra during your last trimester and for just after, when your milk comes in post-birth, you will want to keep the band size and just go up one or two cup sizes to allow for enlarging breasts and room for nursing pads.

We should check our bra size at least once a year anyway because our bodies are constantly changing. As you get back into an exercise routine, finish nursing (if you do choose to breastfeed) and lose your pregnancy weight, your bra size will change again. I know it can seem like a bit of a pain to keep getting measured, but it's important you have the correct support, especially post-pregnancy, and of course as you get older things are starting to slide south, so prevention is the key here too.

You can measure yourself at home, as I said, but I always recommend you double-check by visiting a measuring expert. Most good department stores have trained staff on hand and private measuring rooms. A correctly fitted bra ensures comfort and your clothes will look better, too. There is nothing worse than an ill-fitted bra under clothes with either the breasts bulging out or a big gap between breasts and bra. I've seen many a beautiful dress or top ruined by the wrong bra. Once you make the effort to do it right, you'll be amazed you were ever lazy about it!

The basics of a well-fitted bra are:

* the centre of the bra, in between the cups, lies flat against the chest;

* your breasts should not be spilling out on the sides or top;

* the back band is straight across, not riding up;

* the straps don't dig into your shoulders, nor are they doing all the work.

Common bra mistakes:

* many women wear too loose a band size or too small a cup size – you'll know the cup size is too small if your breasts are spilling out over the top and sides of your bra;

- if your bra looks bumpy or wrinkly under clothes, you should try and go down a cup size or get a good quality T-shirt bra;

- if your underwire pokes you and the wires are coming up too high under your arms, your cup size is probably too big. During and post-pregnancy you will probably be most comfortable in a wireless soft-cup bra;

- if your band gets tighter and tighter throughout the day and you can't wait to take it off, you probably need to go up a size, especially if you are already on the loosest hook;

- bra straps that don't adjust properly can leave you with straps that fall off and become too loose, which is very annoying. Alternatively, you might feel they are always too tight. Either way is giving incorrect support, so be sure to check properly and try on before you buy.

If you are insecure about back fat - which is one of our top body hang-ups according to surveys - and always get a bulge above and below your bra band, try a bra that is specially designed to smooth over these bulges. There are many to choose from on the market now, including bras that have amazing back-smoothing technology that helps to eliminate lines and bulges for the perfect silhouette. Look for bras with higher back and side panels. Spanx have an amazing range and have designed a bra, the

Top tip

Bra-llelujah!, for this very problem. A smooth camisole over your bra and under your clothes works a treat too and will make your outfit look properly gorgeous.

Top tip

Nursing wear

If you are breastfeeding, you will obviously need nursing bras. Again, ease of use and comfort are the key concerns when buying underwear at this time. Nursing wear has come a long way over the past 10 years and there are now lots of options available to you. As your baby will want to be fed when out and about, choosing clothes with easy access is really important as well as bras that you can easily unhook and re-hook singlehandedly.

One of the most ingenious, and yet oh so simple, products on the market for nursing mums is the breastvest (www.breastvest.co.uk). This wonderful invention allows you to wear all your own clothes and still feed discreetly. It's a vest with supportive straps, but the top of it comes to just under the nursing bra. This means it keeps your post-natal tummy under wraps when you lift up your top to breastfeed. Like I said, ingenious! It means you can feed comfortably and discreetly, with no skin on show, and it also saves you money because it cuts out the need for specialised nursing tops.

When I was nursing, I loved and lived in breastfeeding dresses. They are specially designed to offer you convenient access for breastfeeding your baby while on the go, and there are some really nice ones around that are comfy and figure-flattering. Check out www.cherishme.ie, which has a great range that includes Boob and Serafine, and also www.mamalicious.com.

Nursing covers

There are some great nursing covers available and some women prefer these to dressing options. I did use them in the beginning when I was uneasy and getting used to feeding. However, I found that sometimes they can draw more attention to you, plus James absolutely hated having his face covered. Again, this depends on personal choice, comfort levels and the society you live in. When I fed James in a café with a good feeding top no one noticed, but when I had a nursing cover over the two of us, everyone noticed.

I would say, though, that nursing covers are great for first-time mums who feel a bit insecure and conspicuous, like I did, but as your confidence grows and you become more adept at feeding quickly and quietly, you might not need it or want to use it. I did find the covers handy for travel, however. I used mine whenever I was on an airplane, because sitting so close to other people I always worried about making them feel uncomfortable. I do know and understand the argument about feeling free to feed in public, but sometimes it can just be easier to avoid confrontation and negative comments. I'm not saying that's right, but it does make life easier for yourself and your baby.

Breastfeeding in comfort!

* If you are considering breastfeeding, buy a feeding bra during the last trimester. It will save you some money (because if you don't buy a feeding bra and then you decide to feed, you will have to invest in one when the baby is born meaning twice the cost) and will ease you into the transition from pregnancy to breastfeeding.

- Start off with one or two nursing pieces to get you started and as time goes on you can always buy a few more styles to complement your wardrobe.

- Breastvest or similar will save money and help to make you feel more confident.

- Good nursing nightwear is also essential as you do not want to be struggling in the middle of the night when you are already tired. I would recommend Mothercare and www.cherishme.ie for good quality options.

- If you are in any way worried or embarrassed about breastfeeding in public places, use a nursing cover to provide full coverage while you are feeding your baby.

The celebrity post-baby body: reality versus perception

It's normal to be self-conscious about your body after your baby is born, so accept that this is likely to happen and take steps to help build your confidence. Yes, your body has just done an amazing thing, but it's a big change when you go from pregnant body to post-birth body. When you're pregnant, it can often be very freeing – your body looks exactly as it should look. But once the baby has been born, women can feel under a huge amount of pressure to spring back into their pre-baby shape. That's a big ask because you've come out of nine months of radical changes. Why should there be a quick fix?

I know that, post-baby, fashion and my new body had a huge effect on my emotional wellbeing. My body image had probably always been a bit askew considering I started working as a model in Paris at just 16 years of age, but no matter what our circumstances may be, one thing is for sure: our confidence can take a terrible blow as a new mum, so you need to work on building it back up.

Most of us, especially during our teenage years, go through periods of insecurity and sometimes we carry these issues with us into our adult life. Through media and our circle of friends it's easy to become, and remain, obsessed with our body image and to create unrealistic expectations for ourselves. It's no different for pregnant women. We are bombarded with images of bump-tastic actresses and models who, days after giving birth it seems, look absolutely amazing. It's hard to keep focused on reality when you're made to feel inadequate, like every other pregnant woman on the planet is achieving the body beautiful within days or weeks of giving birth. The truth, of course, is that an awful lot of these celeb pictures (if not the vast majority of them) are airbrushed because it's their job to look good and present a certain version of themselves. I'm incredibly lucky that when I did photoshoots after I had James, I had a hairdresser and make-up artist come to my house and I can tell you, it makes a world of difference.

> "There is a very simple golden rule here: don't compare yourself to anyone, especially celebrities."

The other thing to remember is that celebrities have chefs, personal trainers, make-up artists, hairdressers, personal assistants, nannies, night nurses and all sorts of other help, so it's impossible and completely ridiculous to compare yourself with this privileged lifestyle. I know if I had my meals cooked and help with babysitting and a trainer to kick my butt and motivate me, things would certainly be a hell of a lot easier. Add to this a great stylist who will pick flattering clothes to help them dress their new body and hide any lumps, bumps and insecurities they might have and, hey presto!, they are camera-ready.

It's all too easy to get lost in the world of comparison, but it's the equivalent of getting caught up in a world of imagination and make-believe. Comparing yourself with anyone for any reason will drive you crazy. Be inspired by people, sure, but own your own truth and be the best that you can be.

How about some reality checks to put the celeb or model body in perspective:

- only 5–10% of all women are within the height and weight range of catwalk models;

- just about all images in magazines nowadays are altered. In fact, I have done shoots where my own family have failed to recognise me in the final photos;

- even models have really bad hair days, you just don't see them;

- perfection is sold to us daily, but it doesn't actually exist.

The reality is that there are some women who will have bodies to die for even after having a baby, and that's life. Call it genetics, luck or whatever you want, they just slip back into shape really quickly and effortlessly. In reality, these mums are few and far between and most women find it hard in the early days, weeks and months after giving birth, no matter who they are, to accept their new body and feel really comfortable with it.

What's considered beautiful changes from country to country and person to person. We all have our own eyes, so use them to look and think deeper because real beauty comes from within. The most important lesson I learned from spending over half my life in the modelling industry is that nice girls became even more beautiful in my eyes, but beautiful girls who were mean instantly became ugly.

Get to know and love your new body

Self-confidence is not something that everyone is born with, but the great news is that you can work on it and increase it at any stage in your life. If you have never had it before, you can start to work on it right now.

One of the things you'll notice about confident people is that they always have positive role models in their lives who display and encourage self-confidence. They have learned how to be confident because of positive experiences in their lives and a stream of small successes, which then build into bigger successes. We can all create that positivity for ourselves. Find good role models and learn from them. Be inspired by others and heed the wise words of Henry Ford: *Whether you think you can or think you can't, you're right.*

It starts with your mindset. Time for you to do some work! Write down 10 things you like/love about yourself. It can be as simple as:

1. I have nice eyes;

2. I like my smile;

3. I have great legs;

4. I have shiny hair;

5. I have full lips, great hips and fantastic boobs!;

6. I love my shoulders, they are strong;

7. I love my cheekbones;

8. I love my collarbone.

9. I like that I am a kind person.

10. I admire my resilience in difficult situations.

No matter how hard this is, I want you to do it. If you are struggling to do this, then try and think of any time in your life that someone gave you a compliment, like 'your eyes are really pretty' or 'I love your hair like that', 'blue really suits you'. Write each one down and read them back and say, *Thank you.*

Don't ever be limited by the negative things you have been told.

Now, write another list of realistic goals you would like to work on and try to focus on how you want to feel as well as how you want to look, so for example:

1. I would like to feel healthier;

2. I would like to feel confident in a yoga class;

3. I would like to look good in jeans and feel confident in them;

4. I would like to be happier and more content in the body I have;

5. I would like to learn about eating well so I can feel better.

It's important to be realistic with your goals otherwise you will keep setting yourself up for disappointment. It is not humanly possible to lose 10 lbs in a week, but you can lose 2 lbs in a week. You can and will achieve your goals once you allow for the fact that it will take time. As happiness and confidence is an inside job, you need to work from within. So feeling more comfortable in your own skin will give you the confidence to try new things, which in turn will start giving you the results you want.

We all want to look our best, but we absolutely must feel our best too. Changing your body image means changing how you treat your body and yourself, which will change how you feel. It is all linked, no matter how much we try to separate each area of our lives. We cannot treat the mind, body and spirit separately because they are one and when we break a link to one, all the other parts suffer too. This is why eating well, exercising and reducing stress through mindfulness and meditation are really important.

If you eat better, exercise regularly and treat yourself well in thoughts and actions, your skin will glow, your hair will shine and you will feel motivated to live a healthier lifestyle. The natural side-effects of a healthy lifestyle are: vitality, a healthy weight and body size for you, better skin, hair, teeth and nails and overall improved happiness and confidence. What's not to love?!

The key thing to remember is that a healthy body is not linked to one type of body size. In fact, healthy bodies come in all shapes and sizes. Changing your body image means changing the way you *think* about your own body. You won't get anywhere if there is a constant stream of verbal abuse in your head directed at your body. This sort of self-hatred is very harmful – it leaves you depleted and hurt and often depressed. It's very important to get your thoughts working for you, rather than against you.

Don't panic after a baby because the more you panic, the more negative feelings will come up and negative feelings encourage negative behaviour patterns. You need to stop the cycle before it takes hold of you.

Top tip

So one side of the coin is being kind to yourself and thinking positively, and the other side is making healthy lifestyle choices. Together these changes will improve your body image. What are the key lifestyle choices you need to make happen in your life?

* Healthy eating can promote healthy skin and hair, along with strong bones.

* Regular exercise has been shown to boost self-esteem, self-image and energy levels.

* Getting plenty of rest, even with a new baby, is one of the best ways to reduce stress.

Don't replace feelings with food

When you are tired and have crazy hormones running wild after having a baby, it's easy to try to cope with those rampant moods and emotions through food. If your confidence is low, you might feel like you don't want good food, like you simply just don't care. It will be necessary to break this cycle if you want to feel better about yourself both inside and out.

I think every woman knows what it's like to use food as a crutch, we've probably all done it at some stage in our lives. While the junk food and chocolate and snacks might seem great on the way in, the truth is that this can also be another subconscious way of punishing ourselves, without even realising it. For years I used food to fill any uncomfortable gaps. Food was my friend when I was lonely and feeling down. After James was born and my life was so different and so intense, I would binge on sugar in an effort to make myself feel better. It just made me feel worse in the long-term.

The most important thing is how you feel in your own body, and we need to make the connection between food and feelings.

Bingeing on bad food creates a negative self-image because you always feel bad afterwards. As you move towards self-love and self-care you will want to make better choices, and this will happen gradually. But I promise you, once you get on track, you will never look back.

How to get back on track!

* Take baby steps to better food choices. Don't expect to transform your eating in a week.

* Keep a food diary to help recognise when you reach for food.

* If you feel low, try going for a walk or try meditation.

* If you feel low, turn on some music and have a home disco (this actually works and it's fun).

* Keep good food close at hand, in temptation's reach!

* It's never too late to start again – dust yourself off and climb back up on the wagon.

* Enjoy your life and have your treats – just not a week's worth in an hour.

Affirmations

When I was really struggling with my confidence down through the years I started to use daily affirmations, and I find they really work. The key is to keep them simple and try not to overthink them. So choose an affirmation every day as a new mum and say it loud and say it proud – or, alternatively, just say it in your head!

My top 12 daily body image affirmations for new mums

1. My body deserves love.
2. I don't want to look like anyone but me.
3. I love and respect myself.
4. My body is a gift.
5. I've just created a miracle.
6. I'm celebrating me.
7. Beauty comes in all shapes and sizes.
8. I feel comfortable in my own skin.
9. I am much more than my appearance.
10. I embrace my flaws because no one is perfect.
11. I nourish my body daily with great food.
12. I am so grateful for what my body has given me, so thank you, body.

It is vitally important that you watch how you speak to yourself and every time you catch a negative thought popping up about yourself, replace it with a positive one.

A good mantra I use is:

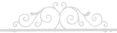

Stop – Catch – Change

Stop your negative thought,
catch it and
change it to a positive one!

This might seem unnatural and incredibly hard in the beginning, but I promise you this will become easier and easier with time. Building good self-esteem means appreciating yourself and treating yourself with compassion.
Keep it simple, keep it real!

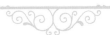

In the first days and weeks we're trying to be everything to everyone, and the sense of responsibility for this little person can be huge. If you have a few friends with kids and babies, support each other and encourage each other and you'll have a much better chance of achieving your goals.

Baby steps are key!

* The first thing to remember is that there are no shortcuts.

* Give yourself a break and be proud of what you've done, mum! Stop comparing yourself to other mums and celebrities. No one can look like someone else, but you can be the best you that you can be.

* Your body needs time to heal and recover and it is not normal to be back in your pre-pregnancy jeans after a few weeks.

* Don't pack away your maternity clothes. Wear them and be comfortable in the weeks post-birth, especially if you've had a C-section.

* Don't try on your pre-pregnancy clothes until you are pretty sure you have a chance of fitting into them, otherwise you'll send yourself scuttling to the biscuit tin for solace.

* Do not diet. I hate that word and I wish we could remove it from our vocabulary. It immediately makes us feel deprived and in want of something to make-up for it. Just make healthy eating habits your eating habits – for life.

Eat energy-rich foods, unprocessed foods and avoid sugar. If you are a mum who is sleep deprived, sugar will mess with your moods and with your hormones. Combining sugar and post-birth craziness is definitely not a good idea.

Go for a walk in the early days and keep it simple – it's a walk, not a marathon.

If you are nursing, invest in some good nursing tops and bras and make sure you are comfortable in them and competent at using them before you try breastfeeding in public. A few private rehearsals will settle your nerves!

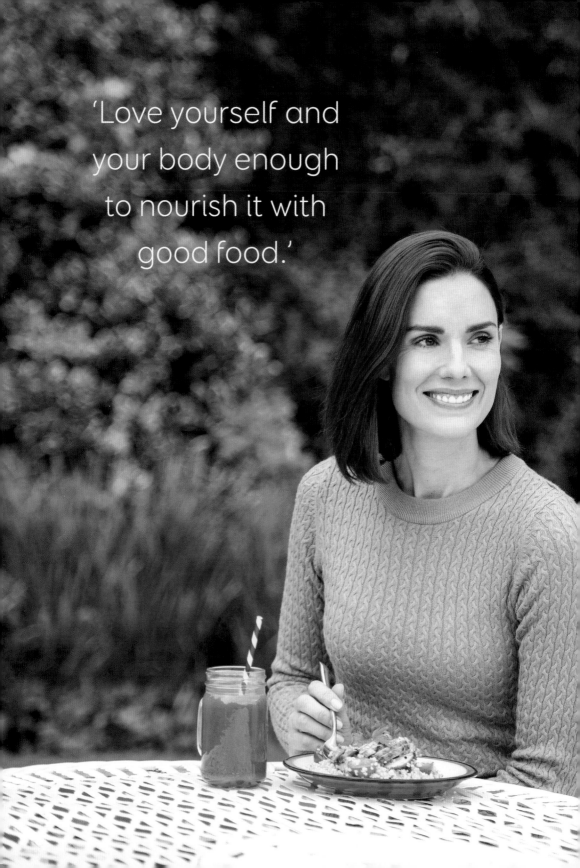

'Love yourself and your body enough to nourish it with good food.'

NUTRITION

5

I want to start this all-important chapter by pointing out that this is an incredibly complex area, with lots of conflicting views and opinions. I have studied Nutrition at third-level, so I have a solid basis of knowledge, but it is also the case that new studies are being conducted all the time and sometimes they contradict earlier studies. It was a curse for us students: something that was true in 2013, say, might be dismissed as untrue in 2015. This means it can be hard to be 100% definitive about these things. But all of the things I'm going to tell you in this chapter come from my own studies and research and, most importantly, from my own personal experimenting and failing and succeeding. This is all based on first-hand experience of nutrition, so I'm passing on my own tried-and-tested methods.

Our food, what we eat and how it makes us feel, is an incredibly important part of our lives. I eat to live, I don't live to eat, and there is a major difference between those two ideas. Some people see food as something they have to do but have little time for. In offices all across the land, people eat at their desks while staring at screens. People stuff food in their mouths, trance-like, while watching TV and if you look around when you are sitting in your car in traffic, you will often see the same thing happening. Skipping meals is common, particularly among new mums, and this wreaks havoc with blood sugar, mood, hormones, sleep and overall general health and wellbeing. For so many people food has become a mindless time-filler, an emotional crutch and an inconvenience.

How our food is made has also changed. When our grandparents were young, all their food was local and fresh. There were no GMOs, nasty pesticides and most people cooked at home from scratch. We, on the other hand, are in an age of fast food, processed food and heavily preserved food, with lots of additives, colours and flavours to enhance the taste and flavour and to prolong shelf-life.

We have moved very far away from a love of simple food and it's telling on our bodies. We need to reignite our love for food and our understanding that it nourishes us at a very basic cellular level.

Think of it like this: when you eat, it is like delivering a very special parcel or present to yourself – something you have always wanted. Inside your body, your cells are super-excited about this and can't wait to open their gifts. When they open their gifts, they are so happy they want to share them with their cousins in every other part of your body. Your body then begins digesting and sorting all of your food into smaller presents of nutrient parcels, and these are sent by special delivery to their new homes where they are needed throughout your body for nourishment, making you feel strong, healthy, satisfied and energetic.

Now I want you to imagine that you have just ordered your dream product, something you have wanted for a long time but couldn't get. On delivery day you open your present eagerly, but it is damaged and broken in parts and you are really disappointed. This is how your body feels when you feed it bad food instead of good food. When we feed ourselves heavily processed, packaged foods, some of the ingredients are unrecognisable to our bodies. When we eat these foods and they are broken down and shared with the rest of our cells, it makes our cells wilt a bit and makes us feel sluggish, tired, moody and irritable.

> *I am not an advocate of a particular type of diet and I am not into extremes. I believe in balance. In my own life, that has been proven to work best of all, so I can stand over it as a reliable and healthy lifestyle choice.*

So my rule is keep it simple and give your body great gifts every day and your body will reward you well. Make choices based on how you want to feel. Do you want to feel healthy and full of life or do you want to feel low, bloated, tired and sluggish? We always have choices in life and like all other choices, this choice is down to you.

I have always loved my food and some of my earliest memories are of my Uncle Noel, who is a chef, making incredible meals, including the most divine birthday cakes you have ever seen. My Nana is also a great cook and growing up I enjoyed traditional Irish food like coddle, stews and, my favourite, a good Sunday roast. My Nana is probably one of the only people left in the Dublin area who still has fresh local food delivered to her door from a family that have been delivering produce for generations.

I am a child of the late 1970s/early 1980s and I ate a lot of junk food growing up. So did everyone else. We devoured cheap penny sweets that were all the rage and chewy bars like Wham! bars that nearly took your teeth out (and I have the fillings to prove it!). As I entered the world of modelling at the age of 15, I saw first-hand how food can be abused and treated like the enemy. I don't even think I heard the word 'health' in the industry in those days. It was during this time, through loneliness, that I became a comfort-eater myself and ate in secret. (It had to be secret because our agency would come and check what we had in our fridges in the models' apartments.) I am blessed that weight never became an issue for me. I would bloat and experience ill health in the form of digestive issues and mood problems, but thankfully I could still work. Having spent over half my life in the fashion industry, I am determined to help people understand that food is good, in fact food is great and not the enemy as so many of us women think it is. It is the type of food you eat that will determine things like weight gain. In fact, we all need to eat less but eat more nutrient-dense foods, to get back to eating a more plant-based diet that revolves around leafy greens and a wide variety of coloured fruits and vegetables. Eating more nutrient-dense foods also ensures that your calories go further.

So here is our first golden rule of nutrition: stop dieting and stop using the word diet.

Before we even begin to talk about the type of food we should be eating for good health as a mum, I want you to remove the word diet from your vocabulary. If I use the word I will be using it to describe foods you should be including in your general diet, not as 'a diet', and there is a big difference!

The reason I want you to do both these things is because diets do not work, plain and simple. The cycle of dieting just messes with your metabolism. Here's what happens when you diet:

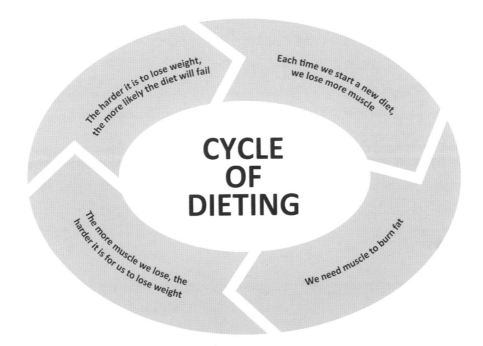

CYCLE OF DIETING

The harder it is to lose weight, the more likely the diet will fail

Each time we start a new diet, we lose more muscle

We need muscle to burn fat

The more muscle we lose, the harder it is for us to lose weight

If you allow it, the cycle of dieting will continue to go round and round, with you caught in the middle unable to jump off.

Dieting immediately makes us think we are denying ourselves something that gives us pleasure. The word diet makes people feel like they're about to embark on a journey of suffering and they usually wake up feeling hungry and salivating miserably at any and all food that crosses their path. To be honest, I have never seen happy people on diets. They are counting calories, days, hours, minutes and seconds until they can go back to their old way of life, which is exactly what got them into the situation of feeling they needed to diet in the first place. The result of this will be failure. Moderation is key and also satisfying your cravings so that they don't turn into binges!

We need to change how we think about diets, food, treats and our lifestyle in general. When you are on a diet, foods are forbidden and because you are human, you will then want those foods more than ever before. I'm not a big fan of cakes, but if I was told that I couldn't eat any cakes or biscuits for six months, I know I would start dreaming about cakes and biscuits all the time. I would walk past bakeries and stare longingly through the window and all the lovely cakes would be staring back at me saying, 'Eat me'.

People diet for many reasons, but primarily to lose weight and feel better about themselves. Nearly all women go on a diet for their wedding, for holidays and special occasions or to lose their baby weight. But instead of torturing yourself, I want you to rethink your relationship with food. Finding balance and harmony is much better for your long-term health and happiness.

I adopted the 80/20 rule a few years ago and it has enabled me to finally find balance, which helps me to stay on track. This means that I am good and I eat well 80% of the time, and for 20% of the time I can allow myself to have desserts, meals out and enjoy parties and events without feeling bad about myself. Nobody is perfect and this rule gives me the ability to be consistent with a clean living lifestyle, which is essential for mood, cravings, weight, energy, health and vitality. This simple rule has finally allowed me to make peace with myself about food, get results and feel great!

What you need post-birth

As a mum you have spent the past nine months looking after yourself better than ever before and now that the baby is here you need to continue to nourish yourself and keep hydrated, particularly if you are breastfeeding.

Here's another golden rule for you: build a healthy lifestyle, don't follow a diet.

I don't recommend supplements as a rule, unless you are lacking something important in your diet and you are medically advised to take them. However, I would recommend staying on your pre-natal vitamin for up to six weeks post-birth (always check with your doctor). Your pre-natal vitamins are more suitable than regular multivitamins because they're high in folate, or folic acid, which some breastfeeding mums lack.

Always check the quality of your supplements and look for those that contain a minimum of binders or fillers of any kind. Tablet-form supplements contain these, so liquids or powders are good. Terranova, Purium and Eskimo are three excellent brands I use, but top of my recommendation list in this regard is Terranova pre-natal vitamins because they have folate in its natural form. I'll let the owner of Terranova Nutrition, Stephen Terrass, explain it as he does it so well:

> 'Folic acid is basically a synthetic version of the folate that is found in foods. Folic acid is not found in nature, and the human body cannot use folic acid as it is – it must first be metabolised into its active methylfolate form in order to provide its benefits. However, recent research has uncovered a shocking statistic that between 9 and 15% of the population have a genetic mutation which significantly impairs their ability to metabolise folic acid. In addition to this mutation impairing the health benefits of folic acid, folic acid which cannot be metabolised properly is thought to build up in some people, leading to toxicity.

When we became aware of just how prevalent and how significant this genetic mutation was, we immediately scheduled the removal of standard folic acid from ALL of our products which contained it and replaced the folic acid with methylfolate, the form which is already active and is not affected by this mutation. As far as I know, we were the first major company in the UK and Ireland to replace folic acid with methylfolate in all products. Not surprisingly, this issue takes on special significance in pregnancy because of the proven role that folate status has in the prevention of neural tube defects.'

The most common complaints post-birth are exhaustion and mood swings and believe it or not eating the right foods can help combat these conditions. You need foods that help with healing and recovery too, so eating a lot of anti-inflammatory foods is important along with fibre-rich foods to help with bowel movements.

In the early days you will need some support and help to get organised. Let friends or family members do your shopping so there is healthy food to hand. Make friends with your freezer! If you weren't close before, having a baby is the perfect time to work on that relationship. Cook in bulk before the birth and freeze enough for the first two weeks.

You don't need fancy ingredients to make food fun; you just need a bit of imagination and variety. I have a food chart with all different coloured fruit and vegetables on it that I use at home for myself and my son. Every day we put stickers on what we eat, with the aim being to get as many stickers on as many different colours as possible each day. It's fun, simple and very effective.

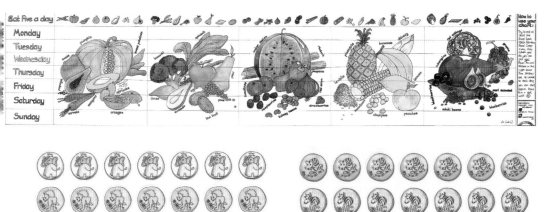

(Source: courtesy of www.lizcookcharts.co.uk)

Let's look at bread

Before we look at all the wonderful things we should be eating everyday, we need to have a word about bread. Irish people adore their bread, but it can become too dominant in the diet, which isn't good. The other problem is that choosing bread can be confusing and some labels are about as credible as politicians. The key to making a good choice is to understand that the first few ingredients listed on any label tell the real story. By law, all food companies must list ingredients in descending order, based on how much they weigh, so for bread you should always look for the words 'wholemeal flour' as the first ingredient on the package, and preferably as the only flour listed. Wholemeal means the flour is made entirely from the whole grain, not just part of it. 'Wheat flour' or 'enriched bleached flour' (or similar) are types of white flour that have much of the fibre and other nutrients removed.

Most grains today aren't 'whole' and some loaves labelled 'wholegrain' or 'wholewheat' don't contain any wholemeal flour (see realbreadcampaign.org for more information). 'Brown bread' is generally made from white flour with caramel or molasses added to make it look dark and healthy. 'Multi-grain' just means that different kinds of refined grains may have been used.

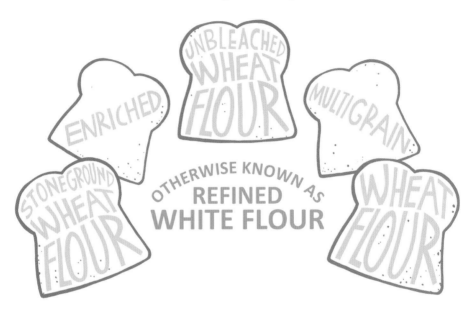

When it comes to bread, wholegrains, aka wholemeal, are what you are looking for because they are healthier. Wholegrains contain all three parts of the kernel. Refining normally removes the bran and part of the germ, leaving mainly the starchy endosperm. Without the bran and germ, about 25% of a grain's protein may be lost, along with numerous key nutrients. Processors are obliged to add back a few vitamins and minerals to refined grains so refined products still contribute valuable nutrients, but wholegrains are far healthier, providing more protein, more fibre and many important vitamins and minerals.

The author of *Healing with Wholefoods*, Paul Pitchford, explains this well:

> *'The grains' protective coating can provide us with a 'protective coating' for improving our immunity and health. Whereas stripping the grain of its coating, through refining essential nutrients out of these foods, strips us of valuable nutrition. If a nutrient starved nation can rediscover the potent value of these grains, a land of excess should soon become a land of moderation and abundant health.'*

So what do we need in our day-to-day diets?

* We need fresh, unprocessed wholefoods. Wholefoods are foods that have either been completely unchanged or changed as little as possible from their original state. Fruits, vegetables, nuts, legumes, fresh lean meats, fresh fish, eggs, dairy – but plain yoghurt as opposed to processed, artificially flavoured ones. 'Wholefoods' is a buzz word and I get that, but if you just try and think when you look at a food that what you want is something that has been almost completely unaltered from its natural or original state. So apples not apple juice, tomatoes not tomato sauce, and things like hot dogs, chicken nuggets and sausages are processed and not fresh! Cheeses, but not the stringy, waxy, processed type. I advise people to stay around the edges of their supermarket (this is true of the layout of most I have been in) and if a food product stays in date for months on end, it is most definitely not a wholefood.

* You need to stay hydrated as most of us do not drink enough fluids throughout the day. There are lots of fun water calculators around now where you put in your height, weight, activity and climate, but again they average out your requirements. Still though, you get a good idea and one thing is for sure: we all underestimate how much water we need. You can eat your water, too. Try not to glug back pints of water in one go, though, and instead spread it throughout the day (the guideline is six to ten glasses for an average person).

Eat fresh and in season food by using a Seasonal Chart

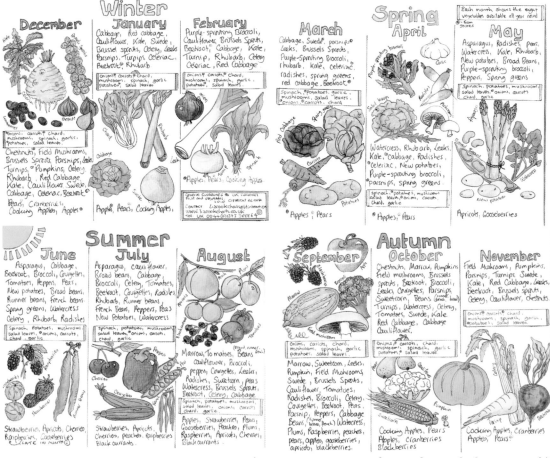

(Source: courtesy of www.lizcookcharts.co.uk)

* Include a variety of different coloured fruit and vegetables, preferably in season, local and organic. (see Seasonal Chart opposite)

* Choose from a large variety of grains and cereals, preferably unrefined as the nutrient content of grains is significantly reduced when refined and processed. So wholemeal breads, oats (porridge), brown rice, bulgar (cracked wheat) are all good. I use barley pearls for soups, even though its jacket has been taken off through a process called 'pearling', which does remove some micronutrients. However, if that outer bran layer is left on, it takes a very long time to cook. Pot barley is the wholegrain version, which you can absolutely use, but you'll just need to be patient.

* Some beans, pulses, nuts, meats, fish, shellfish and dairy.

* The foods that are optional are my '20% foods', which include treats of your choice, and what you like is up to you. I do have to be really careful here because sugar affects my skin, energy, mood and concentration. I have an awful weakness for dark chocolate and if I'm out for a meal, I do allow myself a dessert. My dream is to come off all refined sugar completely as I find once I start eating it, I just can't stop. I am on my way to achieving that goal. Just try and be sensible: for example, a dessert a couple of times a week is fine, but not five or six times! Just always remember you are only fooling yourself and I promise you the cleaner your lifestyle, the better you will feel and you will be less inclined to binge or give in to cravings.

As you can see, we are back again to balance, which is the cornerstone of healthy eating. You need to make sure you are getting adequate amounts of vitamins, minerals, proteins, carbohydrates and good fats in your daily eating.

A good healthy diet is built around fibre-rich vegetables, whole grains, wholemeal breads, pastas, lean meats, eggs, fish, beans, seeds, nuts, fruits, good fats and oils, and healthy beverages (absolutely no fizzy drinks!). A diet low in added sugar will also help you to maintain a healthy weight, increase energy, improve brain function, lower blood pressure, reduce cancer risk and have a more positive lifestyle. The simplest way to achieve this is through consuming a wide variety of foods, which is why I'm a huge fan of the Healing Foods Pyramid because it sets out very simply the myriad choices available to you when you want to eat healthily.

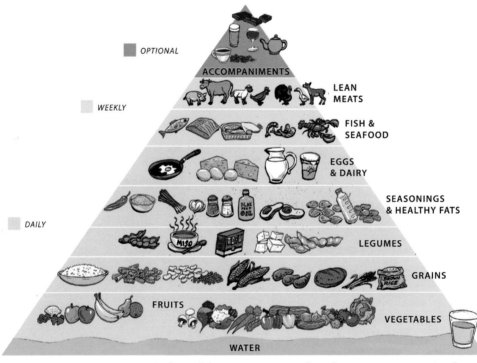

(Adapted from University of Michigan Integrative Medicine:
www.med.umich.edu/umim)

Anti-inflammatory foods

Anti-inflammatory foods can help you to recover from giving birth. Inflammation is a normal and natural response of your body's immune system. However, the trauma and stress of giving birth can sometimes cause the immune system to remain 'switched on' for too long, and this can contribute to a host of health problems. (See my anti-inflammatory juice in Recipes section, p167.) To help your body fight this inflammation you need to consume foods that are considered to be anti-inflammatories.

Examples of anti-inflammatory foods include:

* fennel, carrots, potatoes, butternut squash, broccoli, sweet potato, pumpkin, tomatoes and all green leafy vegetables, such as spinach, kale, collards and mustard greens;

* nuts like almonds and walnuts;

* oily fish like salmon, mackerel, herring (including kippers) and sardines;

* fruits such as strawberries, blueberries, cherries, oranges, pineapples;

* green tea;

* flaxseed;

* spices and herbs such as ginger, turmeric, garlic and rosemary are excellent; cold-pressed olive oil is full of valuable nutrients and other substances with antioxidant and anti-inflammatory effects.

Energy and mood

Your energy and mood after you give birth will be unpredictable and this is down to an erratic schedule, hormones and adjusting to becoming a parent. To help counteract and control this you need to eat often and eat the right foods, which will help to keep your blood sugar stable.

When you are tired all you want is an instant hit of energy, which is why we reach for junk foods and foods high in sugar. Even though these foods can make you feel good quickly, the high is only temporary and you will crash again, leading you to crave more sugar and so the cycle continues. If you skip meals, you will experience a crash in blood sugar and your willpower will fade as the day goes on and you become tired.

A few more golden rules:

* Don't underestimate the power of a single meal and skip meals.

* Eat regularly.

* Avoid sugar and sugary snacks.

Serotonin is a neurotransmitter that helps regulate mood. A meal or snack that contains some protein as well as carbs (sugar/starch) will help to optimise serotonin levels in the brain. So for any new mum, especially in the early days, one of the best ways to fight tiredness using food is to eat small meals that contain protein and carb foods together. This will help both regulate your blood sugar levels and provide enough serotonin.

So here's a quick and simple guide to what is good for you to eat. Enjoy!

* High-fibre wholegrain cereal, such as oats, with berries/raisins and milk of your choice (almond, rice or regular). There are also lots of great sugar-free mueslis around now, like The Happy Pear's version.

* Yoghurt (sugar-free) with sliced fruit topped with almonds, walnuts, or pecans. (Honey, if desired).

* Breakfast burrito (wholewheat tortilla): scrambled egg, mixed veg (peppers, onions) and fresh tomatoes.

* Recently I have found fritattas great when I'm really busy. You can add just about anything you like to them: vegetables like peas, chopped peppers, courgettes and diced tomatoes work great with chopped chicken or ham and a cheese of your choice.

* Chicken salad on 100% wholemeal toast.

* Hummus and wholemeal pitta bread.

* Brown rice, black beans and avocado.

* Broccoli and salmon.

* A lunchtime sandwich of lean meat, either chicken, turkey or beef, on wholegrain bread with a slice of cheese and sliced avocado.

* Pick'n'mixes: go for a combination of dried fruits, nuts and seeds and avoid those with chocolate or added sugar.

* French bean and walnut salad.

* A banana with a handful of raw nuts.

* Fresh vegetable skewers (celery, peppers, cherry tomatoes), hummus, sunflower seeds and wholemeal pitta bread.

* Apple and a nut butter of your choice – my favourite is cashew!

* Cottage cheese with fruit and nuts.

* Chicken and fennel (thinly sliced) in a mixed salad of your choice.

* Plain yoghurt, mixed berries and a drizzle of honey for dessert.

* I also make really quick and easy vegetable soups with lots of different mixed seasonal vegetables and I add in Marigold swiss vegetable bouillion and blitz it in the blender. So simple and nutritious.

* Finally, just a note on the oils I use when cooking: I recommend using coconut oil or olive oil.

A quick and simple guideline for portion sizes

It's very important to watch your portion sizes and not kid yourself about what you're eating.

1 fist = 1 cup (rice, quinoa, etc.)

Thumb tip = 1 teaspoon

Palm of your hand = 1 serving of lean meat or fish

A handful = 28–56 g of snack food (so definitely not 3 or 4 handfuls!)

Depression busters

According to the HSE booklet for new mothers, the baby blues are so common they are considered normal, which leads me to ask: why hasn't it been normalised? Post-natal depression, on the other hand, is when you can't shake those blues and you become bluer. It may affect up to one in seven mums, although some experts believe it affects more. The studies show us that around 13% of new mums in Ireland will suffer from PND, so while there are many lifestyle factors that need to be considered, good nutrition is at the top of my list. I learned this the hard way myself but now, by completely cleaning up my diet, I have finally succeeded in clearing the depression, anxiety and 'brainfog' I laboured under for years. The correct food is a powerful messenger and delivers a message your body needs to hear.

Martina Watts puts it perfectly in *Nutrition and Mental Health: A handbook* and she's worth quoting here:

> 'The handbook for every car manufactured will specify, quite precisely, the grade and type of engine oil that should be used in its engine. Dire warnings are presented as to the inevitable consequences if this advice is ignored, such as loss of power, excessive internal wear, and risk of breakdown.'

She goes on to explain that when it comes to our own bodies, we have completely abandoned any such rationality and thrown away the handbook or simply forgotten there ever was one.

Martina continues on to say that *'we believe that we can fuel a body and lubricate it with whatever we want without regard to any inherent 'design constraints'.'* Most of us also think that there will be no adverse reaction from our bodies or our minds, but really all you have to do is look around to see that isn't true. Depression is at an all-time high alongside the rise in chronic diseases. It's time for everyone to wake up and put the right fuel into our bodies if we want them to work correctly. But we do need to find out what works for us as individuals as we are all different and have different nutrient needs. The only way to do that is by taking control of your choices and seeing which foods suit you and which ones don't.

Zinc

Zinc is needed for hundreds of biochemical reactions in the brain and body and it is important not to be deficient in it, particularly with regard to mental health. A lack of zinc in your diet can lead to irritability and depression. Good sources of zinc include dark-green leafy vegetables (kale, cabbage), pumpkin and sesame seeds, almonds, eggs, fish, turkey, oysters, beef, wheatgerm, yoghurt and wholegrain. (See also Chapter 3.)

Vitamin C

Vitamin C deficiencies have been shown to be linked to depression. Get your vitamin C from citrus fruits, broccoli, green leafy vegetables (especially kale), kiwi fruit, mango, peas (including frozen), raspberries, blackcurrants, parsley, potatoes, spring onions, and turnips. If you've had a C-section or stitches, vitamin C will help you heal. Vitamin C also aids the absorption of iron, which will help with energy levels too. If your doctor prescribes an iron supplement, you need to help your body absorb it. To do this, eat a meal that includes a food rich in vitamin C when you take your iron supplement. It's also recommended to stay away from tea and coffee when you are taking iron as caffeine can impair the absorption.

Calcium

Calcium is actually the most abundant mineral in the body and it plays an important role in maintaining strong bones and healthy blood vessels. Calcium-rich foods may help ward off depression and anxiety. In fact, low levels of calcium may play a role in PMS-related depression, in particular. Your best bets for calcium are green leafy vegetables, almonds, plain yoghurt, cheese, sardines with bones, milk, salmon with bones and sesame seeds.

Folic Acid

Research from Tufts University in Boston, Massachusetts, found that levels of folic acid (folate) were much lower among people suffering from depression than in people who were not depressed. Folic acid in supplements is basically a synthetic version of the folate that is found in foods. Folic acid is not found in nature, and the human body cannot use folic acid as it is – it must first be metabolised into its active methylfolate form in order to provide its benefits. Natural folate is plentiful in avocados, leafy green veggies, beansprouts, bananas, oranges, grapefruit, black-eyed peas, orange juice and most fruits.

Other happy foods include: avocados, bananas, aubergines, pineapples, tomatoes, walnuts and plums.

In the early days it is really important to avoid food that will zap your energy, such as alcohol, poor quality fats and oils, caffeine, white flour products, simple carbohydrates like sugar, and definitely soft drinks.

Constipation

There are so many reasons why you might have trouble going to the toilet after having a baby. For me personally, I was in a lot of pain and I felt very apprehensive even sitting on the loo. If you have stitches and bruising it might even be painful to sit on the toilet, so you could always sit on a soft ring, which I did, and it will help.

The good news is you are not alone and it is actually relatively normal not to do a poo for the first few days.

There can be other reasons for toilet trouble, like high levels of the hormone progesterone in your body during pregnancy, which can cause constipation, plus your digestive system slows down when you are in labour. Some pain relief, like pethidine or diamorphine, could also slow down your digestive system. As you can see, there are many factors that can contribute to constipation and many of them are out of your control. But let's look at what you can do post-birth to help relieve the situation.

There are two types of fibre – soluble and insoluble – and the difference is that soluble fibre dissolves in water, but insoluble fibre does not. So soluble fibre attracts water and forms a gel, which slows down digestion. As a result, it can make you feel full for longer, which can also help control weight.

Sources of soluble fibre include: oatmeal (porridge), oat cereal, lentils, apples, oranges, pears, oat bran, strawberries, nuts, flaxseeds (linseeds), beans, dried peas, blueberries, psyllium husks, cucumbers, celery and carrots.

> *Most importantly, you need to drink lots of water, at least six to ten glasses a day, and eat foods that are high in fibre.*

Insoluble fibres are considered gut-healthy fibres. Most vegetables are known for being high in insoluble fibre, which is a type of fibre that sweeps out your gut like a broom.

If you stir some insoluble fibre into hot water, it won't dissolve; when you stop stirring, it will just sink to the bottom. It will, however, soak up a bunch of the water and expand, the way a dry sponge expands as it soaks up water. Now imagine this puffed-up sponge moving through your intestines and you'll begin to get an idea of what insoluble fibre does for you. Insoluble fibre is a very effective treatment and preventive for constipation and some other digestive disorders. It passes through most of the gastrointestinal tract relatively intact. When it reaches the large intestine (colon) it provides food to the trillions of good bacteria that our bodies harbour there. The more fibre in your diet, the more good bacteria you support in your intestines, and the better your digestion and elimination will work. Essentially, fibre optimises the passage of food and waste through your gut.

Sources of insoluble fibre include: wholemeal bread, whole grains, wheat bran, corn bran, seeds, nuts, barley, couscous, brown rice, bulgur, courgette, celery, broccoli, cabbage, onions, tomatoes, carrots, cucumbers, green beans, dark leafy vegetables, raisins, grapes, fruit and root vegetable skins.

Good sources of fibre include fresh fruits with the skin on, not peeled, dried fruits, vegetables, whole grains such as brown rice and 100% wholemeal bread. Drinking and eating prunes will also help. Prunes were my saviour, and I'm sure all you new mums know what I mean!

To help with constipation post-birth, take a heaped teaspoon of psyllium husks twice daily, just before meals, with lots of water. Linseed/flaxseed are great for digestive problems, too. You can add them to your cereals, like porridge, in the morning and to smoothies.

Top tip

Get your body moving if you are constipated and it will help to get things moving inside. Take a daily short walk in the early days, you might not feel like it, but it will really give you a lift. I also found that massaging my lower abdomen worked well. Try lying down and massaging your tummy (if you haven't had a C-section) and move your legs in to your stomach and stretch them back out again. Trust me, this will help to get everything moving!

(NB: Please speak to your doctor if you are having ongoing problems or if you have haemorrhoids (piles) or fissures.)

Breastfeeding mums

I have never experienced hunger quite like I did when I was breastfeeding. Everyone will be different on this score, but it's generally accepted that breastfeeding uses up plenty of your calories. However, we are slowly learning that we don't need as many extra calories for milk production as was once thought. Your body has stored fat throughout your pregnancy and it will use this for milk production and energy. Isn't nature wonderful!

The biggest mistake mums make when they are breastfeeding is reaching for high-calorie snacks like biscuits that have no nutritional value. Just because you are a breastfeeding mum, it does not mean you can sit on the couch and eat unlimited calories and you'll magically burn them off. The quality of what you eat is also really important for two reasons: your health and your baby's health. As feeding can be exhausting and time-consuming, you will need good quality food that can help build you up post-birth and at the same time ensure your baby is getting great quality milk through you.

Breastfeeding can be a very sedentary activity and a lot of mums will commonly experience ravenous hunger while feeding. As you will be spending a lot of time sitting down when you are feeding your baby, it's easy to fall into the trap of mindlessly eating during this time. If you have healthy food to hand, this will make it easier not to reach for the biscuits. So just as breastfeeding is a choice, our food types and lifestyle are choices too. There is nothing wrong with snacking, I just want you to snack on healthy foods instead of junk. And yes, enjoyable healthy snacks do exist! (See super snacks for super mums on p.161.)

Breastfeeding does not mean you are free to eat what you want. Resist going for the high-calorie foods you would normally stay away from, as you will pay for it later!

A lot of women will lose weight from breastfeeding, but weight alone should not be the reason you choose to breastfeed your baby. Each and every woman's body will react differently to pregnancy. Some women fly through their pregnancies whilst others have problems from day one – they put on excessive weight, have pelvic problems, emergency sections, and the list goes on. The amount you personally need to eat depends on your pre-pregnancy weight, how much weight you gained during your pregnancy and how active you are.

It's not all about food. Remember that you need to make sure you drink enough fluids to satisfy your thirst and that during breastfeeding your body releases the hormone oxytocin, which will also make you feel thirsty.

So what should you eat while breastfeeding?

Keep it simple and choose foods that require little or no preparation. Quick, nutritious foods include fresh fruit, raw vegetables (cut up and ready in the fridge) with hummus, nuts and seeds, melted cheese on toast, cottage cheese, yoghurt with raisins, or sugar-free granola (The Happy Pear in Greystones, Co. Wicklow, has an amazing one).

You don't need to eat anything special or different, just eat a healthy, balanced diet that includes:

- wholemeal bread and brown rice for added fibre;

- plenty of fruit and vegetables;

- some lean protein, like fish or chicken,

- try to have oily fish, like salmon, at least twice a week. (If you don't like fish, see section on Omegas, p.150.)

Eggs are also versatile and quick and easy to cook. Live yoghurt is great, but make sure it has no sugar and add some fruit and honey to taste. You should include lots of leafy green vegetables for calcium and B vitamins and if you find that hard in the early days, make smoothies with your greens. Raw coconut oil (2-3 tablespoons a day) is a must for new mums as it is high in lauric acid, which is a component of breast milk. Lauric acid is a powerful anti-microbial fatty acid that protects the immune system of the foetus and newborn – and don't coconuts look just like our breasts! A Finnish study in 2005 also found that breastfeeding women who consume a diet rich in vitamin C (from food sources, not supplements) may protect their infants from developing atopy (eczema, hay fever, asthma, etc.)

Are there foods you should avoid as a breastfeeding mum?

Most mums and babies do well with most foods, but health professionals are beginning to realise that some breastfeeding infants have a sensitivity to certain foods transmitted via the breast milk. In other words, sometimes babies can react to certain foods in the mum's diet. Experiment if this happens to you and eliminate the suspected food to determine whether the difficulty goes away. In a study (Lust, Brown & Thomas, 1996) in which mums were asked what foods they believed made their babies fussy, they identified broccoli, cabbage, cauliflower, chocolate, cow's milk and onion. But don't be afraid to enjoy highly flavoured foods. If you have eaten them during your pregnancy, the baby will have been exposed to them anyway (see *Breastfeeding and Human lactation/ Maternal nutrition during lactation* – Karen Wambach). My advice would be to attend a nutritional therapist if you are concerned, or contact a qualified lactation consultant like Clare Boyle (www. breastfeedingconsultant.ie).

For me, personally, avoiding alcohol is a no-brainer during breastfeeding, but I wanted to mention it anyway because there are ongoing arguments and conflicting advice about safety and amounts and, of course, everyone processes alcohol differently. Alcohol crosses into the milk and the effect on the infant is dose related. If you want to have a glass of beer or wine, the easiest and safest thing to do is drink it with a meal. (You can subsequently test your milk with a product like Milkscreen, which contains easy-to-use alcohol test strips that will detect alcohol in breast milk). Another option is to pump and dump, but for my money the very best advice is just don't drink alcohol at all.

Caffeine-containing foods or fluids have been questioned before and some mothers do report reactions from their babies, but studies have been shown that the amount of caffeine available to the infant is minimal, only 0.06 – 1.5% of the maternal dose and no caffeine is detected in the infant's urine (Berlin et al., 1984). So if you are ingesting caffeine in moderate amounts, you should be fine. Just remember that too much of anything is bad and moderation is the key.

Hydration

You will never realise how bad you feel until you start to feel good, and dehydration can be the cause of so many illnesses. For the past 15 years I have started my day with lemon water. It all started at a photoshoot one day, when my skin was bad as I suffered with adult acne. A make-up artist told me that drinking warm lemon water every morning would help. It is something that I have done ever since and since studying nutrition I have come to realise that the benefits are far greater than I could have ever imagined. (Drink it through a straw if you are worried about your tooth enamel.)

So my first tip for hydration is to wake up your body with a glass of warm water and lemon each day. (I use half a lemon and a pint of half boiled and half filtered water.) This will kickstart your digestive system and metabolism. It's small changes like this that will make a massive difference to your health. Just think of how dehydrated you are after a night's sleep. Does it not make sense to drink fluids first before putting more food in? When I take a break from drinking warm lemon water in the morning I really notice the difference in how efficient my digestive system is and I also notice a drop in my energy levels. These are the habits I would like you to try for yourself and see if you can notice a difference. Give all these things time. To be honest, it wasn't until I stopped doing it for a while that I started to notice the difference.

Lemons are great because they contain bioflavonoids, potassium and vitamin C. Bioflavonoids are super antioxidants that contribute to good heart health and protect against cancer. Potassium is vital for all cells and tissues, including the brain, as well as helping keep your blood pressure under control. The antioxidants from the vitamin C will really help your skin (healing, especially after a C-section) because it is required to produce collagen, a protein that forms much of the structure of our bodies. Collagen is the framework for our skin and our bones and without it we would quite literally fall apart. Vitamin C also aids the absorption of iron. If you live in a big city, look at vitamin C as a giant antioxidant fire-extinguisher for all the pollution and nasty toxins out there.

Top 10 benefits of drinking lemon water

1. Skin.

2. Weight loss.

3. Immunity.

4. Detox.

5. Iron absorption.

6. Brain health.

7. Antioxidant.

8. Potassium.

9. Bioflavonoids.

10. Heart health.

Why is it so important to stay hydrated?

Water is not only the most important nutrient in the body, it is also the most abundant. Water is critical to the balance of all the body's systems, including the brain, heart, lungs, kidneys and muscles. A 2% drop in body water can cause a small but critical shrinkage of the brain, which can impair neuromuscular coordination, decrease concentration and slow down thinking. Your body depends on water to survive. Every cell, tissue and organ in your body needs water to work correctly. Your body uses water to maintain its temperature, remove waste and lubricate joints.

How does my body lose water?

* Urinating.

* Sweating.

* Breathing.

* Hot weather.

* Exercise.

* Illness – vomiting or diarrhea.

Mild dehydration is one of the most common causes of daytime fatigue and it is estimated that 75% of us are dehydrated in some form. This is very bad news because proper hydration is necessary to keep your body working efficiently and effectively. It helps your kidneys and digestive system to function properly. Most people who complain of constipation are chronically dehydrated!

The effects of dehydration are unpleasant and unhelpful to your body.

* Slower metabolism.

* Fatigue.

* Muscle pain – increase in lactic acid in muscles, increase in blood acidity (causing muscle tightness and increased muscle soreness post-training).

* Thirst: during exercise, sweating releases the electrolytes potassium, sodium and calcium, which are known as electrolytes. There is not much in most types of drinking water, so they need to be replaced. Coconut water or ¼ tsp of Himalayan salt in pre-workout smoothies or juices is a good idea.

* Headache.

* Dizziness.

* Increased heart rate.

> " *Water is the single most critical nutrient. Think of it like this: your body can live for up to 50 days without food, but without water you will only survive for three days.* "

If you're worried about whether you're getting enough to drink, check the colour of your urine. If it's pale-coloured, you're getting plenty to drink. If it's dark yellow or smells strongly, or if you feel lethargic or faint, you may be dehydrated, in which case you should drink more water. You should aim for six to ten glasses per day. Different people need different amounts, depending on your activity throughout the day, but try to tune into your thirst.

Get more water into your day by keeping a bottle with you all the time and by drinking herbal teas (caffeine is a diuretic). Eat your water by including water-rich fruits and vegetables in your diet, like cucumber and watermelon. And remember, if you are breastfeeding, you need lots of extra fluids.

Top tip

Matcha green tea

I discovered matcha green tea when I was recovering from post-natal depression. I have always suffered from anxiety on and off, but this tea has made a huge difference to my life. It helps to calm the nervous system because of its high levels of l-theanine, an amino acid. With 137 times more antioxidants than regular green tea, 70 times the antioxidants of orange juice and nine times the beta carotene of spinach, matcha tea is most definitely in my 'must have' food picks.

I call matcha my secret superpower and I add it to smoothies, juices, yoghurts or I drink it as a shot. It does not come in a teabag but rather as a fine powder, which makes it easy to use in baking and cooking. I mix a small amount into a bottle of warm water and carry it with me during the day to sip on. It also helps to curb sugar cravings so can help with weight loss.

In order to buy quality matcha tea, you need to choose wisely and do your homework. There are a lot of cowboys out there trying to sell matcha cheaply and in bulk because it is gaining popularity. Look closely at the ingredients and on some of them you will even find rice bran solubles forming the bulk of the main ingredients, which you definitely don't want. Only buy top grade, 100% matcha green tea. I buy from www.koyumatcha.com. The yellow is great for anxiety and mood, which is why it's called 'mellow yellow', but the green is great for digestive issues and low energy.

Drinking matcha just once a day is said to boost your metabolism by 35–43% and I always take a shot of matcha before a workout as it can increase fat oxidation (when your body uses up fat stores to produce energy during exercise). Try replacing your morning cup of coffee with matcha and watch your skin, nails, hair, energy levels and focus improve. (Check out my YouTube channel for videos.)

Top 10 benefits of drinking matcha green tea

1. Increased energy levels.

2. Clearer skin and stronger hair and nails.

3. Anti-carcinogen.

4. Lowers blood pressure.

5. Boosts metabolism.

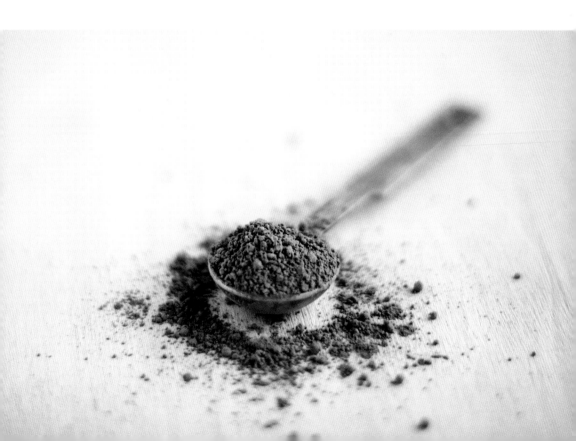

6. Full of antioxidants.

7. Prevents UV damage.

8. Improved memory and longevity (source: http://www.
    matchatea.co.uk/Matcha-Green-Tea-Focus-s/1833.
    htm).

9. Protection against heart disease and diabetes
    (source: http://www.matchatea.co.uk/Matcha-Green-
    Tea-Antioxidants-s/1831.htm and also http://www.
    pacificcollege.edu/news/blog/2014/07/26/green-tea-
    type-ii-diabetes).

10. Anti-aging – the longevity of people in Okinawa,
    Japan, has been somewhat related to their regular
    consumption of matcha green tea.

Omegas

One group that we hear less about is fats, in particular essential
fats, but fat is a very important component of the body, with
60% of the brain consisting of fat and all cells surrounded by a
membrane that consists of fat. We want to keep our cells happy, so
it is important we give our cells enough omega-3 to prevent them
from getting sad.

Essential fatty acids (EFAs) are a crucial part of a healthy diet
because our bodies **cannot** make them. When the word 'essential'
is used in nutrition it means that the substance in question is vital
to our health but that as the body cannot synthesise (manufacture)
it, the substance must be obtained from the diet.

Inflammation is a vital capability of our body – without it we would have little protection against infection and injury. But when inflammation outstays its welcome, it harms our health in a multitude of ways.

Omega-6 and omega-3 oils work together to promote and regulate inflammation. Basically, omega-6 is needed to make inflammation happen, while omega-3 keeps it under control. Both are necessary, but the problem is that omega-3 is very scarce in today's common foods whereas omega-6 is abundant. Inflammatory problems are the result.

You have undoubtedly heard of omega-3 fish oil, which is the omega most people are familiar with because of wide advertising of its health benefits. But did you know that, with over 8,000 clinical trials, omega-3 fish oil is one of the most researched substances in modern medicine? This indicates the level of importance attached to omegas.

Omega-3 (Alpha-Linolenic acid) and omega-6 (Linoleic acids) are used by the body as building-blocks for many of the larger fatty acid molecules vital to our cells. Of special interest are the omega-3 fatty acids EPA (Eicosapentaenoic acid) and DHA (Docosahexaenoic acid). Apart from their role in controlling inflammation, these are essential for the structure and functioning of the brain and for overall health – without adequate amounts, our health will eventually suffer in one way or another.

DHA and EPA are especially abundant in the brain, eyes and heart. Sufficient DHA ensures that the brain, retina and other parts of the nervous system develop properly, while EPA seems to be particularly vital for the healthy functioning of these and other

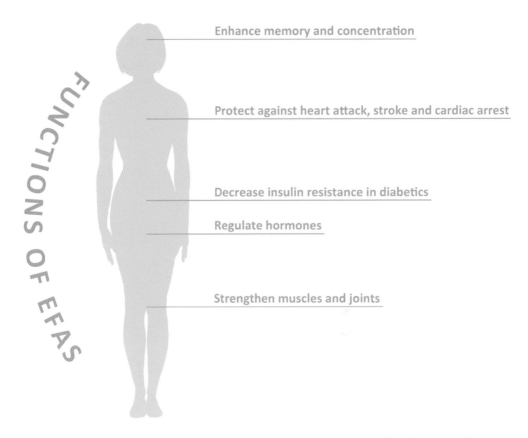

FUNCTIONS OF EFAS

Enhance memory and concentration

Protect against heart attack, stroke and cardiac arrest

Decrease insulin resistance in diabetics

Regulate hormones

Strengthen muscles and joints

tissues throughout the body. As DHA is important for brain and eye development and function throughout life, it is important for breastfeeding mums to ensure they are getting enough.

The evidence that omega-3 delivers major health benefits is very clear, but let's look at it a little closer.

Essential fatty acids (EFA) have many roles in the body, with involvement in two main areas: cardiovascular health; and brain and nervous system function. While both omega-3 and omega-6 are essential, they are not created equal. The main goal of using omega-3 fatty acids is the reduction of inflammation. EPA is the most effective of the omega-3 fatty acids in reducing inflammation and because omega-6 fatty acids tend to promote inflammation, achieving a good balance is key.

The omega-3 oils EPA and DHA can be found in oily fish, such as salmon, halibut, herring, mackerel, oysters, sardines, trout and tuna (fresh), while the plant omega-3 occurs in flax and chia seeds, walnuts, hemp and some types of microalgae. Omega-6 is abundant in eggs, poultry, mayonnaise, cereals and vegetable oils. A healthy diet needs to contain a balance of omega-3 and omega-6 fatty acids, but these days we have too much omega-6 in our diets and too little omega-3. Research indicates that the ideal ratio of omega-6 to omega-3 is between about 2:1 and 4:1. But a typical US/western diet has … wait for it … a ratio between 10:1 and 30:1!

Because EPA and DHA can also be made from ALA, the omega-3 fatty acid that is found in high amounts in flaxseeds and chia seeds, this is where vegetarians and vegans should go to get their omega. However, it is important to know that the conversion of ALA to DHA is very inefficient and for this reason vegetarians and vegans are often lower in DHA than meat-eaters. It is now possible to buy supplements containing vegetarian DHA, sourced from algae.

Docosahexaenoic acid (DHA) is an essential omega-3 fatty acid found in fatty fish and fish oil. It is also found in microalgae, which is a suitable dietary source for vegetarians.

Top
tip

In order to optimise your body's supply of essential fats rich in EPA and DHA, aim to eat oily fish – such as salmon, mackerel, sardines, herring, anchovies and fresh tuna – at least three times a week.

> **"** *Less than 10% of flax omegas get converted to EPA and DHA, which is why fish oil is nature's best source of omega-3.* **"**

Eskimo-3, which I use, derives oil from sardines and anchovies. These are small fish, so their bodies have less time to accumulate pollutants, such as mercury, in the water compared to larger fish, such as tuna. Tuna should really be limited to twice a week. I used to eat canned tuna four times a week until I did my research. (If you'd like to read up on this, check out http://www.env-health.org/IMG/pdf/5-_Mercury_and_Fish_Consumption.pdf.)

Omega-3 fatty acids have been shown in numerous clinical studies to combat depression as well as bipolar disorder (see *Nutrition and Mental Health: A handbook*, Watts), and I absolutely believe they played a big part in my recovery from post-natal depression. Research has shown that women who suffer with post-natal depression produce breast milk that is very low in DHA. Basically, the baby's needs are greater than the mother's and it uses up her stores. It is recommended by the European Food Safety Authority (see http://www.efsa.europa.eu/en/efsajournal/pub/3840) that all pregnant mothers take an omega-3 supplement in the form of DHA during pregnancy and while breastfeeding. This will ensure that mum and baby get their essential fat.

Flaxseed and flax oil are a good source of omega-3 ALA (Alpha-Linolenic Acid). The main problem with ALA is that it must be converted into EPA and DHA in order for your body to benefit from the good effects attributed to omega-3s. As I have said before, this conversion process is not very efficient, with as little as 10% being converted to EPA and DHA. Although flaxseeds (and flax oil) and chia seeds are inferior to fish as sources of omega oils, they are great for digestion, hormonal health and for the skin. For this reason I add flaxseeds to porridge and smoothies.

Vegans can get this important fatty acid by taking algae supplements.

I know I've said that I'm not a supplement pusher, but I feel very strongly about omega-3. If your diet is lacking in something as important as omega-3, then you need to either eat oily fish (salmon, sardines, mackerel) two to three times per week, or supplement with a high-quality fish oil, such as Eskimo, to boost your levels. It's that simple!

It is more important than ever to make sure you are getting enough omega-3s as our western diet is really high in saturated and trans fats, which can cause inflammation, contributing to inflammatory conditions such as arthritis, eczema, heart disease and inflammatory digestive disorders. Omega-3 is nature's own powerful way to combat inflammation.

As I said previously, our omega-6 consumption has increased dramatically over the last 100 years. This is due to an increased consumption of vegetable oils, grain-fed livestock (no longer free-range), decreased wild game consumption and processed foods. As omega-6 can cause inflammation, too much omega-6 knocks our system off balance and it's important to redress that balance. If your only way or best way to do this is through supplements, then so be it. Omega-3 is so important to your health, it's worth it.

The following could all be signs of fatty acid imbalance:

Dry, unmanageable hair	Dry skin
Excessive thirst	Dandruff
Brittle, easily frayed nails	Frequent urination
Hyperactivity	Irritability
Dry eye	Behavioural disturbance
Learning problems	Soft nails
Poor wound healing	Allergies
Frequent infections	Lowered immunity
Patches of pale skin on cheeks	Weakness
Cracked skin on heels or fingertips	Fatigue

What does omega-3 help to prevent and treat?

Alzheimer's disease	Diabetes
Arthritis	Heart disease
Asthma	High blood pressure
Attention Deficit Hyperactivity Disorder (ADHD)	High cholesterol
	Obesity
Breast, colon and prostate cancers	Osteoporosis
Burns	Schizophrenia
Depression/bipolar disorders	Skin disorders
	Stroke

Source: *Fats that Heal, Fats that Kill,* Udo Erasmus (Alive Books, 1993); and *They are what you feed them,* Dr Alex Richardson (Harper Thorsons, 2010).

Vitamin D

Vitamin D is the only vitamin that the Irish government stipulates must be taken in supplement form between 0 and 12 months. (See *Vitamin D supplementation for Infants – Information for Health Professionals and Policy on Vitamin D supplementation for Infants in Ireland*, both reports published by the HSE.)

Vitamin D is essential for the absorption of calcium. The link between vitamin D and strong, healthy bones was made many years ago when doctors realised that sunlight, which allows you to produce vitamin D, or taking cod liver oil, which contains vitamin D, helped to prevent a bone condition in children called rickets. Rickets is a defective mineralisation of bones due to deficiency or impaired metabolism of vitamin D and has been rearing its ugly head again in recent years, with the number of cases here in Ireland on the rise.

Vitamin D is the sunshine vitamin, so there are no prizes for guessing why we don't have enough of it in Ireland. Some studies have suggested that the overuse of sun cream is also partly responsible for the growing number of cases of vitamin D deficiency. You don't need to tan or burn your skin to get vitamin D. You only need to expose your skin for around half the time it takes for your skin to turn pink and begin to burn. How much vitamin D is produced from sunlight depends on the time of day, where you live in the world and the colour of your skin.

Vitamin D is essential for healthy bone development and is really important, especially during pregnancy, for new mums, babies and toddlers. Recent research has shown that vitamin D may be important in preventing and treating a number of serious long-term health problems and is also really important for the maintenance of healthy bones and teeth, immune system, muscle function and brain development.

As vitamin D is essential for the absorption of calcium, it's important for all mums, whether breastfeeding or not, to ensure their baby has enough vitamin D. If your baby doesn't have enough, it won't absorb enough calcium from the milk it's being fed to enable it to build strong teeth and bones. Accordingly, the advice here in Ireland is to give your baby vitamin D supplements for the first 12 months at least.

The winter months can be really hard for a lot of people, so if you are a winter new mummy, then vitamin D is really important. The days are shorter, some people start to feel a little sad and it's also the dreaded 'flu season. One of the things we do have control over, however, is making sure we are getting the nutrients we need and eating a good diet.

It is usually estimated that about 40% of people are deficient in vitamin D, but it is in fact more in the region of 40–75%, which is quite shocking. (This information is contained in an article (http://www.webmd.com/food-recipes/guide/are-you-getting-enough-vitamin-d) and in a website (www.vitamindcouncil. org) dedicated to vitamin D research.) Those most at risk are old people, babies and pregnant mums. Some of the symptoms of deficiency are vague and can include tiredness and general aches and pains. Some people may not have any symptoms at all, so please check with your GP if you have any suspicion you have a deficiency and a blood test can be done to check. Both James and I take a supplement, as I know for sure we don't get enough sunlight.

One of the most interesting new research studies has found that vitamin D supplementation in pregnant mothers and subsequently in their newborn infants may together reduce the risk of developing acute respiratory infections. Acute respiratory infections (ARIs) refer to any infection in either the upper or lower airways. ARIs are common in children under the age of five, with an average of three to six cases per year; with our damp weather, our babies can be prone to respiratory infections.

Vitamin D receptors in both the immune and respiratory systems indicate a direct role for vitamin D in these systems. And vitamin D could play an even more important role during pregnancy and infancy with regard to the development of a healthy immune system and respiratory system. (For the latest vitamin D news and research, visit www.vitamindcouncil.org.)

When it comes to successful and healthy nutrition, it's all about balance!

Every time we open a newspaper or turn on the TV and radio we are getting mixed messages about our food, so here are my top tips for keeping it simple.

My top tips for keeping it simple:

* eat seasonal fruits and vegetables (for very helpful charts, see p.123 and p.126 and www.lizcookcharts.co.uk);

* eat whole foods;

- buy organic when possible;

- spend more time in the fruit and vegetable aisle in the supermarket;

- cut down dramatically on sugar;

- cook at home when possible;

- make friends with your freezer and cook in bulk;

- enjoy your food;

- don't eat pre-packaged/processed food/ready-made meals;

- don't eat any food if you can't understand the ingredients;

- if your grandmother used to eat it, it's good!;

- eat a large variety of colours;

- mix it up daily – having variety makes it less boring;

- eat 100% wholemeal bread instead of white bread;

- never underestimate the power of a single meal (so don't skip meals);

- have fun with food!

The Recipe Section

Now we get to put all that research and information into practice, with yummy results! This section aims to make it easy for you to start making changes. Take it bit by bit, choose one change at a time and focus on it for a week, then move on to the next change. This way, you won't overwhelm yourself with a grand plan, therefore you're far more likely to succeed. The goal, and the reward, is a healthy diet and lifestyle that benefits your body – and your family's bodies – in every way.

Super snacks for super mums

You should keep snacks simple and tasty so they are tempting and easy to prepare. Here are some good ideas:

* nuts: small portions (handful) of unsalted raw nuts;

* two Japanese rice crackers with a nut butter of your choice;

* hummus and vegetable sticks (carrots and celery);

* small plain Greek yoghurt with berries and seeds;

* coconut milk yoghurt – CoYo (www.coyo.co.uk);

* smoothie (see Smoothies and Juices section, p.164);

* vegetable chips/crisps with curried yoghurt and fresh mint (add ¼ teaspoon curry powder to 4 tablespoons of plain yoghurt);

- oatcakes with nut butter and sliced banana;

- wholemeal bagel with ricotta and strawberries drizzled with honey;

- chopped avocado with chopped cucumber, squeeze of lemon and pink Himalayan salt (pink Himalayan salt has trace minerals you need after birth and for general good health);

- salad with sliced tomatoes with goat's cheese and pine nuts;

- small wholemeal pitta with tuna, salmon, chicken or cottage cheese;

- small salad with chicken, fish, chickpeas or a hard-boiled egg;

- apple slices sautéed in coconut oil and sprinkled with cinnamon (great winter warmer);

- 2 cups chopped watermelon, 25ml fresh lime juice, large pinch Himalayan sea salt and 4 tsp cayenne pepper – blend with ice and it's amazingly refreshing;

- apples with almond butter;

- scrambled egg on wholegrain toast for a snack packed full of protein and energy;

* lettuce wraps: you can fill them with almost anything, chicken salad and cheese, or goat's cheese, pomegranate and chicken;

* pomegranates can liven up any salad – here are my favourites:

  spinach, pear and pomegranate
  fig and pomegranate with mixed greens
  chopped kale, orange slices, pomegranate and walnut
  pomegranate, feta and beetroot

* with regard to salads, I always make my own dressing with two parts olive oil to one part balsamic vinegar, squeeze of fresh lemon with cracked black pepper and a touch of pink Himalayan salt; and I always add sprouted seeds (see Smoothies and Juices section, p.164);

* avocados with Herbamare or pink Himalayan salt (I never use regular salt anymore as this has more minerals in it!) and a sprinkle of chilli flakes on crackers;

* healthy snack bars with absolutely no sugar, like those made by Bounce, Nakd, The Primal Pantry and Creative Nature, are all great for mums on the run. But beware of so-called healthy snack bars that are loaded with many different forms of sugar, including glucose syrup, invert sugar syrup and much more.

Flavoured waters

Yes, we can even make water fun! I like to make a big jug of flavoured water and leave it in the fridge overnight. You can add cucumber, apple, citrus fruits, mint, basil, berries and much more. And remember to squeeze some extra juice in, as well as the fruit pieces!

My own tried-and-tested favourites are:

* lime and mint;

* mixed berries and basil;

* medley of citrus: orange, lemon and lime;

* mint and cucumber.

Smoothies and Juices

I juice and blend at home and as a busy mum my blender has been a lifesaver when I don't have time to juice in the morning – plus it's so easy to clean. I add a scoop of coconut oil to my smoothies for a healthy fat boost and this makes a great snack, especially for new mums in the early days.

The question everyone asks, of course, is whether there is a difference between juicing and blending. The answer is: yes, there is.

The main difference is that juicing removes the pulp and extracts most of the liquid nutrients and water from the fruits and vegetables. Blenders, on the other hand, pulverise the whole produce, making it into a smoothie. The pulp is what is called indigestible fibre (we encountered this earlier), which has no

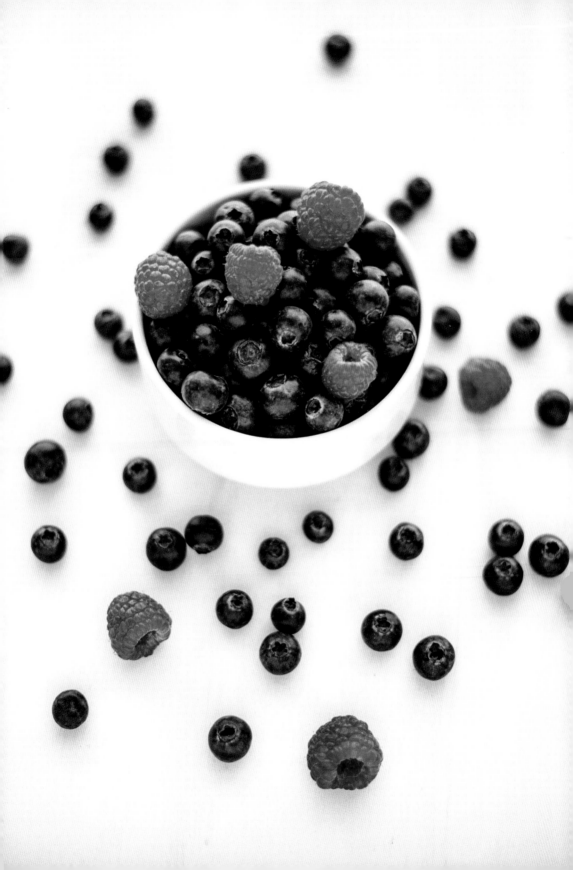

nutrient content but is essential and very important for a healthy diet. It helps to keep your digestive system and gut healthy and it also slows down the absorption of sugar, which is why you should not juice a lot of fruits together as the sugar will get absorbed quite quickly and your blood sugar will become unbalanced, leading to mood swings and, believe it or not, energy loss.

The trick is to use mostly vegetables (80%/90%) when juicing or blending. When I'm juicing, I always notice how much more produce I go through, which means that a glass of juice has more vegetables in it than a same-sized smoothie. As Jason Vale, the master of cold-press juicing, says, juicing really is 'a nutrient express'. My son James prefers juices because he doesn't like the consistency of the smoothies, so again it all comes down to personal choice.

Juicing and blending is fun and it's a great way to use up fruit and veg that's about to go bad instead of wasting it. I'm going to give you some of my favourite recipes in this section, but you'll have your own favourite and least-favourite fruit and veg, so experiment and find out what sets your taste buds zinging. Personally, I don't use many fruits except berries. I tend to eat oranges whole, because I like to get the fibre, and eat fruit salads instead of juicing them. But the absolute key for me is the amount of veg, particularly green vegetables, I can consume in juices or smoothies. It's much more than I'd manage if I had to eat it steamed or cooked.

Juices for minding mum!

My favourite post-birth anti-inflammatory juice is a simple carrot, apple, beetroot, ginger and turmeric juice. This is a powerful antioxidant and anti-inflammatory drink full of vitamins and minerals to help the body heal post-birth. This combination has also been touted as a powerful cancer-fighting juice. I find it very hard to get enough veg into my day sometimes, especially when I am busy, so this is a great way of making sure I'm getting a lot of nutrients.

Tame the flame

6 small carrots

2 red apples

1 fresh beetroot

½ inch of ginger

1 inch of turmeric root

I put the smaller items, like the ginger and turmeric, in between the larger items to juice!

Top tip

Another great anti-inflammatory juice is my

Green Goddess

Large handful of kale or spinach

½ cucumber

3 stalks celery

1 green apple

¼ pineapple or a small cup of pineapple chunks

2 inches of ginger

½ lemon

Constipation buster

In the early days you want to help your bowels as much as you can by including ingredients like psyllium husks in your diet. But psyllium husks alone with water is tasteless and boring, so here is a great juice to liven it up.

> ### Get moving and grooving, aka apple, carrot and cucumber juice
>
> 2 apples
>
> 4–6 carrots (depending on size of carrots)
>
> ½ cucumber
>
> 1 tsp of psyllium husks and 230–300ml of water or coconut water
>
> I juice the apple, carrot and cucumber and then I add them to the blender with the psyllium husks.

(Note: I also find pure fresh orange juice great for constipation, too.)

Energy and immunity

'Eat your greens!' How many times have you been told that since you were a kid? But because the idea of eating a whole lot of greens can make our stomachs turn, we end up leaving out an important source of what I like to call the little soldiers that fight hard against just about every toxin, free radical and chronic disease marauding about the place today. Greens also help boost immunity, protect against cell damage and are very low in calories. In other words, they are your best friend! I cannot tell you how having green smoothies has changed my life and

I know that sounds dramatic, but it's true. They take little or no time to prepare and my energy and mood and concentration are much improved.

I like to stick to greens (40–50%) for the basis of most of my smoothie recipes. I generally tend to use either kale or spinach as the base (sometimes kale can be a little bitter, though, so again it's up to the individual). Then I add:

1 small avocado

1 tablespoon of Supergreens (all good health food stores have them)

¼ cucumber

1 tablespoon coconut oil (optional, but recommended)

Big sprinkle of mixed seeds or sprouts (Seeds are great for getting your omegas. Omegas are good fats essential for our brain, heart health and general health and wellbeing – see section on Omegas, above.)

Fill to the line with almond/rice milk (if looking to lose weight or you don't like almond milk, use water or coconut water)

You can buy Supergreens in any good health food store. I usually throw a scoop in to bulk up the nutrient content even more because Supergreens are foods that are incredibly powerful in the fight against chronic diseases, immunity, inflammation … and the list goes on!

I also use a lot of sprouted seeds, which I buy online from The Happy Pear (www.thehappypear.ie). They can be used in smoothies, salads and sandwiches and wraps and they are packed with nutrients. You can get a mix of broccoli, alfafa, clover and radish, and their bean mix is great too.

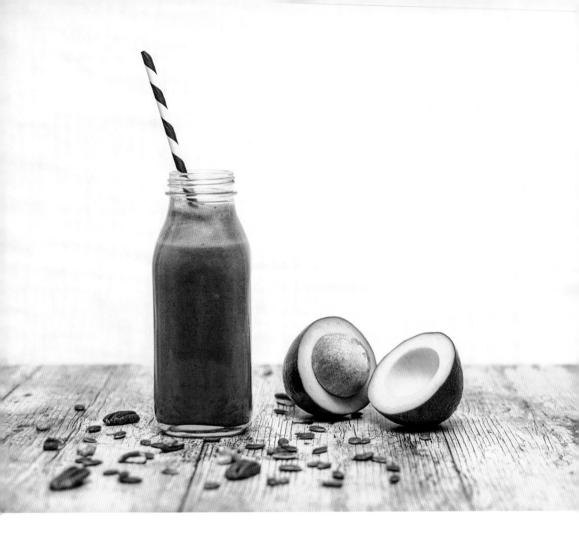

I also make wheatgrass shots at home. It's simple, nutritious and packed full of goodness. In my opinion, it is nature's finest medicine.

The one thing I do love about blending is that I can throw in extra greens and supplements and things like seeds to add extra nutrients and I find I'm then much fuller and more satisfied on the run. I love using avocados as they make the texture creamy and delicious.

Here are some extras I add in:

mixed seeds, including pumpkin, sesame and chia

sprouts

mixed beansprouts

matcha

maca powder

spirulina powder

Life Drink (from Terranova), which is an intensely nourishing blend that contains a staggering array of health-promoting ingredients. It gives you the ideal and optimum nutritional balance to help your body perform at its very best. Most good health food stores stock it.

If I'm hungry in the morning and feeling a little down, I know I need energy and all the nutrients that my body is craving. I used to skip breakfast, but now I make smoothies on the run and take them in the car. So for this next Energy and Immunity recipe I put in a lot of seeds because omegas help with my mood. I also add an avocado for more good fats and energy and some oats, as they are a slow-release form of carbohydrates (you can also use gluten-free oats). I also add a big cup of frozen blueberries as they will give your antioxidant levels a boost for the day.

So for a boost to energy and immunity try:

Morning Motivator

1 cup of oats

1 scoop of Life Drink (Terranova)

1 small avocado

Huge sprinkle of mixed seeds

Large cup of frozen blueberries

Fill to the line (blender) with almond milk

The berries should make it sweet enough for you so you don't have to add any sugars, even in the form of honey!

Sometimes I mix it up between juicing and blending to make a combi-drink, and this one is particularly delicious:

Pick-me-up

I first juice the beetroot and three carrots in the juicer, and then into my blender I put:

Large handful of kale

Juiced beetroot and carrot

¼ cucumber

Handful of mixed seeds

1 scoop of Supergreens or Life Drink (Terranova)

Fill to the line with filtered water

This smoothie is also great for weight loss for new mums!

Slim and Sassy

Small handful of kale

2 small florets of broccoli

¼ cucumber

Tablespoon of mixed seeds

Tablespoon of chia seeds

3 sprouts (seasonal) or sprouted seeds (small handful)

1 stalk of celery, chopped

½ lemon without the rind (you can also use lime)

1 large scoop of Supergreens

Fill to the line with water or coconut water

(Note: I like to use pretty much all veggies, but I know when my friends come they like me to sweeten up the juices for them. So if you are not used to green drinks, you can add a small bit of pineapple or a ¼ to ½ of an apple or some red grapes to sweeten. You can also add a small handful of frozen mixed berries (which I buy fresh and freeze). I would love you to work towards having mostly vegetable smoothies and juices and if you persevere, your taste buds will change with time, I promise!)

I place all my ingredients for one smoothie in individual freezer bags and prepare my drinks for a week. All you need to do is take the bag out of the freezer, empty contents into the blender, add water, blend and a cool refreshing smoothie awaits!

Top tip

Another great brekkie on the run for a busy mum is:

Breakfast in one or on the run

Small cup of oats

Small handful of mixed seeds

1 frozen banana

Small handful of mixed frozen blueberries and raspberries

Fill to the line with almond milk

 I buy my berries fresh and then freeze them as warm smoothies are not very tasty. It also means I don't have to worry about the fruit going off.

Antioxidant powerhouse smoothies

This smoothie is packed full of hard-working soldiers called antioxidants, which help fight off free radicals. Antioxidants work hard every day as one of the first lines of defence the body uses to help prevent cell damage. We need to keep our army strong!

Defence Force

Large handful of kale

Scoop of Supergreens or Life Drink (Terranova)

Small handful of frozen blueberries, blackberries and raspberries

1 stalk of celery, chopped

1 tablespoon of coconut oil

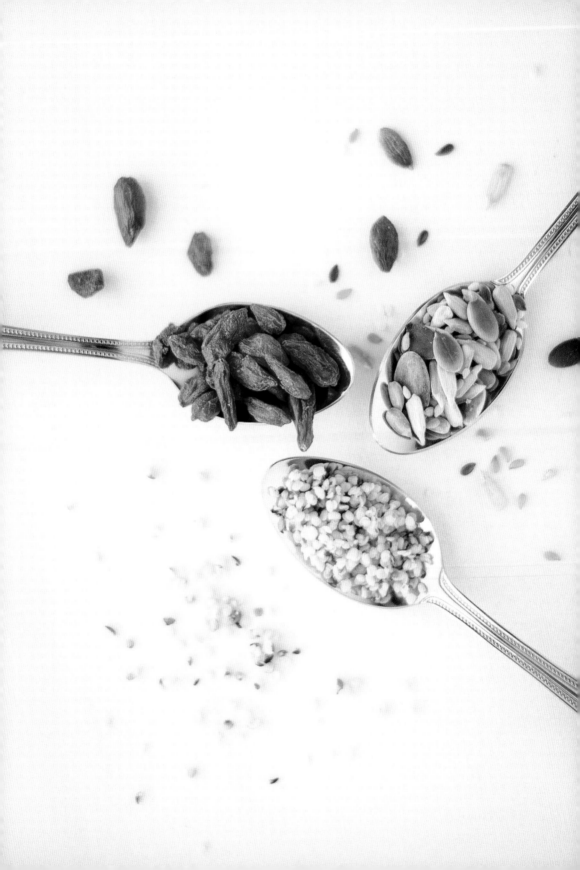

Fill to the line with almond milk (it's also nice with just regular or coconut water)

If you want to be a little more adventurous, there are lots of great ingredients and products on the market that you can try, such as chia seeds, goji berries, hemp, cacao and mulberries. I find they add a delicious flavour, and cacao is amazing mixed with frozen bananas and almond milk if you are looking for a treat!

Spirulina Surprise

Handful of spinach

Scoop of spirulina

1 small avocado

2 frozen bananas

Fill to the line with ½ almond milk and ½ coconut water

 Top tip If you don't like avocados, replace them with other greens, like broccoli, spinach, celery or even apples.

It's a good move to add spirulina to your diet. The United Nations has declared spirulina the best food for the future as it is one of nature's most potent and most nutrient-rich foods. It is a complete source of protein, containing every essential amino acid that our body uses to build healthy muscle and tissue, and is also rich in essential fatty acids as well as the B vitamins, Beta carotene and chlorophyll, which cleans the body. Its boosts immunity and has been shown to help fight against allergies too. In other words, a super-soldier!

MY TOP FOOD PICKS

THE FOOD	THE REASON
Cherries	Rich in antioxidants that can help fight inflammation. Drinking tart cherry juice has been shown to reduce inflammation and to aid sleep as it's full of melatonin.
Salmon	Rich in omega-3 fatty acids, which help lower blood pressure and inflammation, reduce the risk of heart disease, stroke and cancer and help balance mood.
Green leafy vegetables	Great anti-inflammatory foods and the more you eat, the better your body's ability to heal. Eat lots of salads, especially during the summer. They are high in B vitamins, including folate, which remain important vitamins even after birth for healing and breastmilk supply. Greens also contain vitamins A and C and K, which help fight infections and also helps with blood clotting and healthy bones. Greens also contain iron, zinc, calcium, magnesium and other trace minerals. What's not to love!
Avocados and Avocado oil	A rich source of healthy fats, which help lower bad cholesterol. They contain nearly half your recommended fibre intake and are a rich source of potassium and vitamins K, B9, B6, B5, C and E. Avocados are also great for your skin, help to balance hormones and help improve circulation (See Chapter 7, p.225).

Plums	A post-natal superfood, helping to ward off post-natal depression. They boost immunity and have great healing potential, helping to prevent inflammation and infection. I love to dice them up and add them to salads or mix them with plain yoghurts.
Lentils	Versatile, can be pre-made and are great for bulking up soups and stews in the winter months. They contain the detoxifying and antioxidant powerhouse selenium (of which Brazil nuts are the top source), which is one of the few nutrients in breastmilk that does depend on the mother's dietary intake because, just as in pregnancy, all other nutrients will be taken from the mother herself!
Sweet potatoes	Full of calcium and magnesium, which are known to be 'calming minerals', so these are great to help reduce anxiety post-birth, especially in the early days. They also contain vitamin C, which means they promote immunity and healing. Bake them and add shredded ginger to boost the immunity even more.
Bananas	I love bananas because they are convenient, full of vitamins, minerals and fibre and they have an incredible array of health benefits, including being an anti-depressant, aiding sleep and digestion and being a great source of energy. Perfect all round, then!

Quinoa	Quinoa is quite new on the scene but very versatile and easy to cook. It dates as far back as the Incan civilisation and believe it or not the Incas recognised the value of it as an aid to conception. The called it the 'mother grain' and offered it to gods in ceremonies. It is rich in B vitamins and minerals, folate and zinc. It can be eaten hot or cold. I add it to salads and you can sweeten it and have it in the morning as porridge!
Coconuts and coconut water	I absolutely love coconut oil and because it is mainly composed of medium chain fatty acids (or Triglycerides), which are easily digested and sent straight to the liver for energy production, it means it is not stored as fat and can actually can help boost your metabolism. I use it in smoothies and cooking and also in my beauty routine (see Chapter 7). You do need to make sure you are buying a good quality, raw, organic, virgin coconut oil. If you struggle with the taste in cooking, you can buy a mild, odourless version. There are plenty of good brands around now. I use Coconova, Biona or coconut water, as long as 100% coconut water is the only ingredient listed.
Apple cider vinegar	The list of benefits derived from drinking it is impressive. It is used to treat tummy trouble, hiccups and bad breath, prevent indigestion, clear sinuses, boost energy, aid weight loss, control blood sugar, boost immunity, decrease cravings, treat a cold, it has anti-fungal properties, helps with allergies, asthma and regulates PH level in the body. It helps dissolve kidney stones, helps with nausea, skin problems and gout.

Nutrition advice for the early days

- Cook in bulk and freeze food.

- There are companies that deliver nutritious meals to your door, such as www.gourmetfuel.com, and this is a great gift for any new mum in the early days.

- Shop online and have it delivered.

- Ask for and accept help from friends and family members.

- Set an alarm on your phone to go off at different intervals during the day with the message: FOOD?

- A bowl of porridge in the morning will set you up for the day. Oats are rich in iron, calcium and magnesium, which are vital for your depleted mineral stores after labour.

- Make life easy and eat nourishing food that's convenient.

- A lot of mums have trouble sleeping because of their new and erratic schedule, so try eating tryptophan-rich foods like bananas, turkey, spinach and eggs. Tryptophan is an amino acid that produces serotonin (see earlier), which helps you relax and feel happy, but these foods need to be eaten alongside carbohydrates to access the brain, so banana and toast is a good combination.

My challenge for you as a new mum is to make one small change to your lifestyle and diet every month and see how you feel. It doesn't sound like much, but that will be 12 improvements in a year. Please don't overestimate what you can do, which is how we often sabotage ourselves and then slip back to our old ways. Small changes over time means that good/new habits become ingrained and you will have a better chance of sticking with them.

I would love for these changes to become rewarding habits as you adjust to your new arrival.

* **Eat mindfully** – this helps in every way as your body is more relaxed and, believe it or not, thinking is actually the first stage of digestion, called the 'cephalic' phase. It sets off a chain of events in your body that gets your body ready and prepped for the digestion process. I'm not talking about taking hours out of your day, I simply mean if you only have 10 minutes, make those 10 minutes count and be present when eating.

* **Start each day with lemon water** and drink water regularly throughout the day as it will help your skin, energy levels and overall health.

- Chew your food properly. Sounds simple, but most of us barely chew our food and this is an important part of digestion, too!

- As much as possible, steer clear of processed sugar.

In the weeks that follow . . .

As your routine starts to settle into a rhythm, continue to mind yourself. Introduce some exercise you enjoy doing and get out and about to mum and baby groups. Continue to accept help as a parent. Be grateful if you have it, knowing that one day you'll return the favour. The saying is true: it really does take a village to raise a child.

Maintenance

Minding mum nutritionally is not a temporary project, it's a lifelong commitment to your own self-love, which I have said many times before and will say many times again before this book ends. Minding mum is selfless, not selfish. Have fun with food and live a positive life and enjoy every second with your kids.

My 10 Golden Rules post-pregnancy

Try these top tips and my handy eating plan to get yourself on track.

1. Get lots of vitamin C for healing, especially post C-section.

2. Support your hormones with zinc (red meat, nuts and seeds, egg yolks and oats) and vitamin B6 (broccoli and bananas).

3. Stay stress-free by meditating, taking a hot bath, doing yoga, or going for a short walk in the fresh air, or something similar you enjoy.

4. Don't set yourself a weight-loss goal immediately post-birth; give yourself a break. Remember that everyone is different and it will take time and you have just created a miracle, so appreciate what you have done!

5. Maintain your blood sugar balance with small meals regularly. Avoid refined and sugary carbohydrates and stay away from diet products as they are simply laced with sugar.

6. Aid digestion with fibrous foods such as fruit and vegetables, whole grains, beans and my constipation busting juice (recipe above).

7. Support your immune system with prebiotics like onions, garlic and rye and with probiotics like live yoghurt.

8. Eat a range of essential fats found in nuts and oily fish to reduce any inflammation (take an omega-3 supplement if you don't eat oily fish).

9. Detoxify your body from chemicals by not smoking, limiting alcohol and caffeine intake and eating organic food when possible.

10. Be kind to yourself – speak kindly to yourself and treat yourself well.

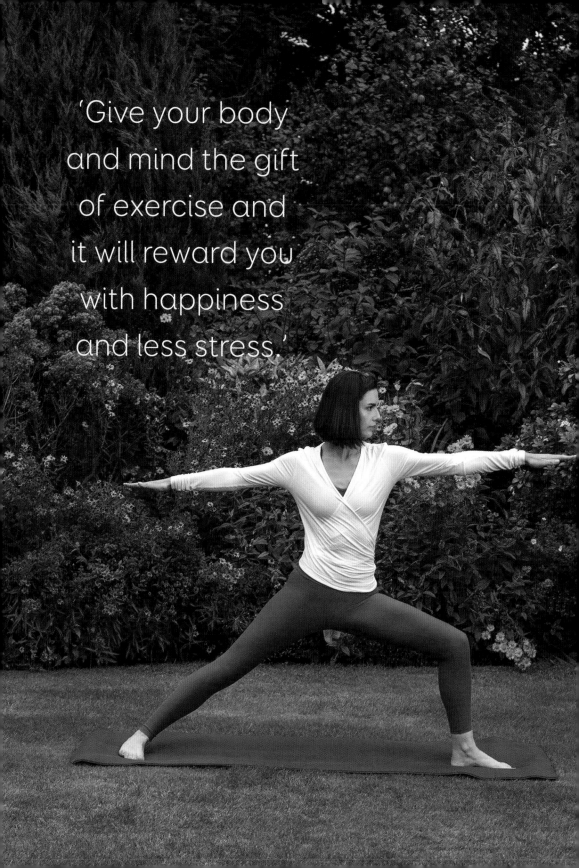

'Give your body
and mind the gift
of exercise and
it will reward you
with happiness
and less stress.'

EXERCISE
POST-PREGNANCY

6

ove it or hate it, exercise is here to stay and we all need it. But let's look at why we need it so badly. Very simply, our health and wellbeing depend on it, and by health I mean health in body, mind and spirit. Exercise serves each of these areas in such a positive way and is the string that ties them all together. You would be forgiven for thinking that exercise is all about weight loss because in the western world it seems as if that is what it has become. We see people being punished and put through their paces in an effort to get results and it all looks very unappealing and hard. Personally, I feel that weight loss is a side-effect of living a healthy lifestyle and for once this is a side-effect you want and need.

If weight loss is your only goal, then most of the time you will be setting yourself up for failure. You will have blinkers on and you will run headfirst into obstacles and dead-ends, usually ignoring all the other areas of your life that need to be worked on simultaneously to help you achieve your goals. If you do this, enough will never be enough.

Most people will also be disappointed with their weighing scales. The scales can change daily due to so many factors, including hydration and toilet habits, but if the scales go up, your mood usually goes down and so the cycle begins. This can be a nightmare none of us needs or wants.

So in order to avoid getting caught in a negative weight-loss cycle, here's what you can do:

- throw away the scales;

- focus on your feelings;

- join the dots within your lifestyle habits and find your own formula;

- nourish yourself with good food, and the bonus here is that you can then eat more of the right thing!;

- find an exercise you **enjoy**;

- be realistic as a new mum and set realistic goals;

- be healthy and happy, not skinny and miserable;

- be good to your body and it will be good to you;

- understand that exercise is not just about weight loss;

- stretch first thing every morning to help reduce stress and start your day the right way.

Find an exercise you enjoy

We are all unique and different, which means we will all have different tastes in food, men, clothes, make-up, jobs, holidays and people. Exercise is no different, so please, ladies, stop forcing yourself to do an exercise that makes you miserable. I've lost count of the amount of mums who tell me how much they hate the gym but they have to do it because they need to lose their baby weight. *Newsflash:* No, you don't! There are hundreds of different exercises out there to choose from, so have fun trying them all out until you find one that suits you.

We need to move away from feeling we have to do things and then doing them and being miserable before, during or after. When you become a mum, time is precious and if you only have an hour maybe once or twice a week, please don't waste it being miserable.

For years I got up at the crack of dawn and went to the gym and mindlessly went through the motions because I felt I had to for my job. The key word here is *mindlessly*, which means I didn't really benefit from it in the ways that I should have. Now that I finally have confidence (after only 30-odd years!), there's nothing I won't try. I run, walk, jog, workout with a trainer, practice yoga and pilates and the best part is, I have fun doing all of it. Sometimes I get to exercise only once a week and sometimes a lot more, which is all part of being a mum. I switch it up depending on how I'm feeling and I don't put pressure on myself anymore. I listen to my body and I always come out with a smile on my face and you can too. Here's how:

> " *Enjoy your fitness journey as this is your life and you need to enjoy it all, not just the end results.* "

* don't take it too seriously and have fun;

* use affirmations silently during exercise or out loud if you're on your own (see Fitness affirmations, p.208);

* don't beat yourself up if you miss a week/class;

* push yourself and try new things;

* congratulate yourself on your achievements as you go, big and small.

As women we spend our entire lives worrying about our weight. We are dictated to by magazines and celebrity culture. No matter what – and believe me I know, I've been in the fashion business for over half my life – we're never happy with the way we look. We've said this before and it's time to say it again: don't compare yourself with anyone else. Learn to embrace and love your body type and know that if you nourish your body from the inside out and exercise regularly, you'll be on your way to being healthy in both body and mind in no time.

Love life, choose an exercise that you like and that suits you and that you will benefit from. There is definitely something out there for everyone. Some people like sticking to the same type and love routine, others like switching it up. Find your happy exercise zone and go for it!

Nature really is truly amazing and from a tiny egg your body has formed a little person! Imagine how much work and just how complicated it is to make organs, bones, and tiny little hands and feet. Phew … I'm tired just thinking about it! I cannot stress how important it is **to give your body a rest** immediately post-pregnancy. Yes, this is a chapter on exercise and how crucial it is, but for new mums adequate rest and relaxation is equally important. It's that old chestnut – balance – that's what you're aiming for in exercise as much as in food.

What happens to your body after you have a baby?

Relaxin

During pregnancy a hormone called relaxin is released that affects post-pregnancy readiness for exercise. Relaxin is a hormone produced by the ovary and the placenta and its function is to 'relax' your ligaments and slacken your joints. This is essential for the bodily changes that occur through the trimesters because it makes the pelvis flexible, which is necessary for giving birth.

While that's necessary in the delivery room, it has an adverse effect on your stability. The down side of relaxin is that it affects other areas, not just the pelvis, so it works on the ankles, wrists and knees, too, for example. And once you've given birth, you don't go back to normal there and then. It takes time for your body to stop producing relaxin and for the effects of it to disappear. The time it takes increases if you're breastfeeding, because your body will continue to produce it. Again, you can learn from my mistakes: I went back exercising too quickly and pushed myself too hard and ended up hurting my knee and wrist, which meant I had to wear supports for the next two years! What I should have factored in was that we are more prone to injury during this time when our bodies are busy growing, giving birth and feeding our babies (and I was still feeding my baby).

Due to the presence of relaxin in your post-birth body it is recommended that you wait at least six weeks before you begin to exercise properly, and that stretches to six to eight weeks if you had a C-section. Most importantly, always check with your doctor before beginning any exercise programme and get the all-clear.

It's highly recommended to wait six to eight weeks before exercising properly after birth. However, I would strongly recommend and encourage you to do Kegel exercises for your pelvic floor and also stretching exercises from the minute you give birth – and with your pelvic floor you can start pre-birth!

I think we really underestimate the benefits of stretching (gentle stretches, especially after a C-section) coupled with breathing correctly (inhale for four counts and exhale for four counts) because it can do wonders for your mind and body. Your mental health is extremely important and delicate at this time, so joining the dots to connect eating well, moderate exercise and resting as much as possible is very important. I stretch first thing in the morning and throughout the day. It's a very simple way to get the body gently moving and it keeps your energy flowing.

I know you've heard this already, but you have to be realistic about your goals. The bottom line is that 99% of mums don't live in Hollywood and don't have access to chefs and personal trainers 24/7. It took nine months to create a baby and it will take **at least** that long to shift the weight gained during that time. It went on gradually, remember, so do not expect it to come off all at once. Crash dieting will damage your metabolism and set you up for a possibly lifelong miserable relationship with food.

There's no big secret to losing the weight and yes, some have to work harder than others, but like anything in life you get what you work for. Being healthy is not just about looking good, it's about feeling good too. With regular exercise you'll sleep better, your mood will improve and your quality of life will get better as a result. These are pay-offs worth working for!

Pelvic floor work using Kegel exercises

Kegel exercises are called after an American gynaecologist, Arnold Henry Kegel (1894–1981). He invented the now famous Kegel exercises, which involve squeezing the muscles of the pelvic floor in order to strengthen them. You need to pay attention to your pelvic floor long before you give birth because a strong pelvic floor will help reduce your risk of incontinence, will boost your core strength and stability and will improve your sexual health which, if we are being honest with ourselves, is what so many women worry about post-pregnancy. I can't tell you how many times I have heard my girlfriends say that they are worried they will never be the same again 'down there'. Let's face it, we all worry about springing back into shape! Well, there's good and bad news: bad news is it will never be exactly the same, but who cares because the great news is that it will be pretty darn close if you do your Kegel exercises and allow your body to heal properly.

The pelvic floor is like a hammock that supports your bladder, uterus, vagina and rectum and when the pelvic floor is weak, all of these areas can't function as well as they should. This is why you need to do your exercises and if you are reading this thinking, *Damn, I haven't been doing mine*, don't worry, just start right now!

One of the key ways to keep your pelvic floor strong is learning how to isolate it so you can give it a workout. Kegel exercises are the squeezing and releasing of your pelvic floor muscles, but there is a right way and a wrong way to do this.

The right way to do Kegels

* First things first, you need to find the pelvic floor muscle. The best way to find it is to try to stop the flow of urine when you are peeing. If you manage to hold back the flow, you have found the muscles you want to target and work.

* Contract these muscles, pulling them up towards your abdomen, and it should feel as though you're squeezing and lifting them slightly up into the body. Just imagine that you are squeezing a small pebble with your vagina – that's the sort of contraction you're looking for.

* If you are having trouble doing the exercises, don't panic. Immediately post-birth you might still be numb

and not feel them, but please ask your doctor or nurse for advice or try doing your Kegels in front of a hand-mirror. If you're doing them properly, your perineum, or the skin-covered area between your vagina and anus, should contract with each repetition.

* Start small and try and do them several times a day – just a few reps each time, holding the contraction for a few seconds, with the aim of building up to holding it for 10 seconds. Take your time and increase them slowly.

* Continue the exercises for as long as it takes to feel comfortable again, which can be several months or more for a lot of women. No harm in continuing anyway as you will only gain from doing them – especially in the bedroom.

I kept forgetting to do my Kegel exercises in the early days and weeks and, let's be honest, we have so much to think about with a new baby that it's impossible to remember everything. But let me tell you, when I sneezed or coughed and leaked, I remembered pretty quickly to do them then.

The beauty of Kegels is that they are invisible, private little movements, therefore you can do them any time, anywhere. You can be squeezing away while:

* standing in the line for groceries in the store;

* sitting watching TV;

feeding the baby;

in the car;

first thing in the morning when you wake;

last thing at night before you go to bed;

at work;

in restaurants and cafés and anywhere else that takes
your fancy!

For women who are experiencing leaking, getting back into serious fitness can be a problem. Just make sure that you are wearing supportive clothing and always wear a sanitary pad when you are working out. If you feel a cough or a sneeze coming on, tighten your pelvic floor; if you are sitting down when this happens, really squeeze to help prevent leaking. EVB compression sports shorts are made specifically for this reason: www.evbsport.com.

Some women will need to do pelvic floor work for a considerable amount of time after having a baby, or indeed forever. If you don't see an improvement and it's affecting your life and your confidence, please go and see a specialist for pelvic-floor physiotherapy. Don't suffer in silence or be too embarrassed to ask for help! This is something that could bother you for the rest of your life if you don't take steps to sort it out.

So, just what exercise can you do and when?

The American College of Obstetricians and Gynecologists (ACOG) recommends that it's okay to gradually resume exercising as soon as you feel you are up to it, but of course this will differ for everyone. If you are fit and exercised throughout your pregnancy and had a vaginal delivery, you can start exercising almost immediately. By exercising I mean a short walk, some stretching and maybe some sit-ups when you are ready. If you had a C-section, your scar will need time to heal and your movements will be limited for six to eight weeks, including driving and most exercise. If you feel up to it, after a few days you can go for a slow walk, but only if you feel up to it.

Of course, with all this relaxin surging through you, you need to be extra careful or you'll end up injured like me. You have to modify your activity and listen to your body – and I mean *really listen*. If you feel something is a potential problem, stop doing it before it becomes a real problem. There is damage you can't undo – like overstretching ligaments. They won't pop back into shape. This means you must take it easy and if your body isn't ready for something, don't force it into submission.

A healthy core means a healthy body

Pregnancy will usually have a detrimental effect on your abdominal muscles, and you'll have to do some work to get them back working at 100% again. If you don't do this, your pelvis, back muscles and spine will pay the price for your abs' laziness. It takes patience and time after pregnancy, and sometimes a minor miracle, to find those belly muscles again, but they are there. They won't like being put back to work, but they have no choice if you are to feel fit and healthy again.

Diastasis Recti

Before you begin any abdominal work you need to assess yourself, or be assessed by a professional, for diastasis recti, which occurs usually during the last trimester of pregnancy when the connective tissue between your abdominal muscles thins, causing your muscles to separate. It is a condition whereby the right and left sides of the rectus abdominis, the so-called 'six-pack' muscles, spread apart at the stomach midline (the linea alba). Believe it or not, it's actually quite a common pregnancy condition, but some women may have a more severe case. If you do, it is recommended to exercise under supervision.

How to check yourself for diastasis recti:

* lie on your back with your knees bent;

* contract your abdominal muscles;

* press your fingers gently into your abdomen above and below your bellybutton;

- inhale, and as you exhale lift your head and shoulders off the floor;

- if you can feel a soft spot or gap between the muscles, then you do have a separation.

- One to two finger-widths is normal and should close on its own. It will take around four to eight weeks for the gap to close on its own.

- If your gap is wider than three finger-widths, you should contact a physical therapist to ensure proper closing of the gap.

- If you start to exercise before the gap closes, you will risk injuring those muscles. (For more information on this, see the Physiotherapy section at http://www.guysandstthomas.nhs.uk.)

I feel you should always err on the side of caution, especially in the early days, and exercise under supervision. But once you're ready to get working on those abs, there are so many mum workout classes now, like www.babybodyfit.ie (stroller-based), where you can join in and bring the baby along and exercise with other mums. You can also try restorative yoga or a gentle mom & baby yoga class or Pilates.

Abdominal exercises

For most women, the tummy is the area of their body they are most anxious about post-birth. Once you're ready to exercise, there are lots of things you can do at home to get you started.

Crunches: these will help to strengthen your abs initially and then you can advance and move on to sit-ups. This might sound old-school, but it's one of the best exercises to get your abdominals into shape quickly.

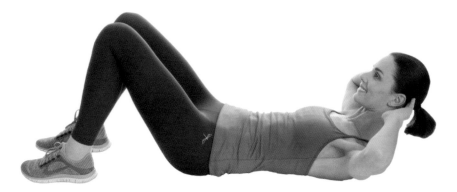

How to crunch: lie on your back with knees bent and feet flat on the floor, with hands behind your head so your thumbs are behind your ears. Crunch up towards the ceiling, then return back to start position. Do three sets of 8–10 crunches to start.

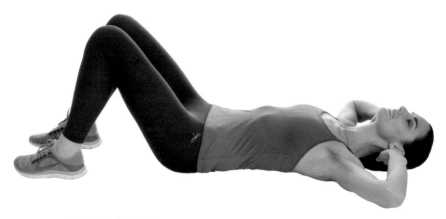

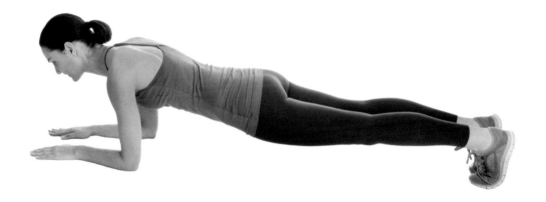

The Plank: this is hands-down my favourite exercise. I absolutely love it as it really gets results and is something I can do every day at home. It can really help you to sculpt your waistline and it also helps with posture, which is important after a baby. Again, start small and do 3 x 10–20-second holds, building continuously as you get stronger.

How to plank: start on your elbows, facing down, and up on your toes with the body held straight in a plank-like position. Ensure that arms are under chest and shoulders. Hold in a static position for between 20 seconds and 2 minutes.

Squats: these will soon tone up your thighs and calves, and if you keep your abs pulled in for the duration, it will benefit your core muscles too.

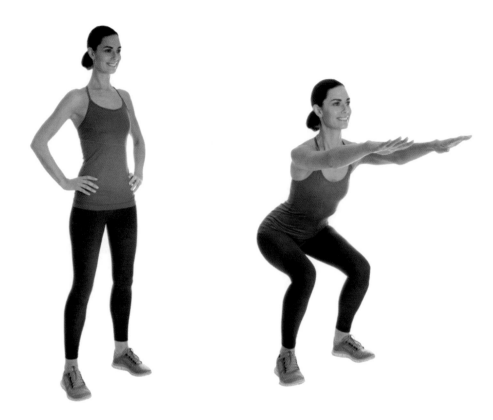

How to squat: stand upright with your hands by your side and your feet shoulder-width apart. Lower your body towards the floor, sending your hips back and down and bending your knees, bringing your arms up to chest height in front of you for balance. Push through your heels to return to start position, keeping your back flat. Do three sets of 8–10 squats.

Lunges: another excellent exercise to tone up and strengthen. This is an essential exercise for abs, thighs and calves.

How to lunge: start with feet shoulder-width apart, then lunge forward with one leg, dropping back knee towards the ground. Push up from the front foot to return to start position and then repeat on opposite leg. Do three sets of 10 on each leg.

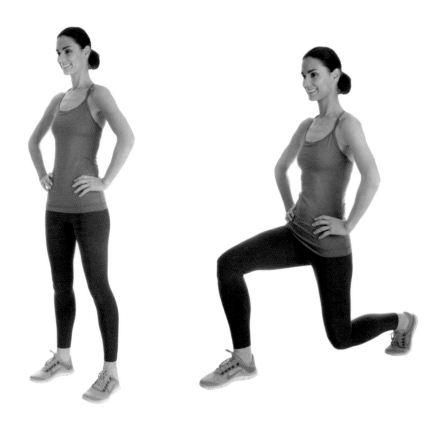

Pilates

Pilates is excellent for both pre- and post-natal fitness. Most importantly for me, it incorporates both body and mind because of the deep breathing it includes. I was blessed to meet Sarah MacLachlann, a Pilates master, who is a gifted teacher and whose mantra is: the devil is in the detail. When I started with Sarah, she assessed my posture, checked for a diastasis recti (separation of the abdominal muscles) and then recommended a few private sessions to start with. In those sessions she introduced me to my pelvic floor and deep tummy muscles, how to do tummy exercises without hurting my neck and back and ultimately showed me how to exercise correctly. Then I was moved on to small group classes. The result? I had reduced back pain and I got my shape back. You can also do mat Pilates classes, which are great, too, but as I have a bad back I find the reformer Pilates more supportive.

Reformer Pilates is done using a machine, which means you have more support as you perform the moves. Pilates can be done on equipment or on the exercise mat. Over the years things like yogalates and modifications have been added, but they are all derivatives of Joseph Pilates' original method. The reason for these variations is to make it fun as Joseph's original version can be quite tough for some people. Over the years people have added in their own modifications, but my advice is to try different teachers and classes until you find a class you enjoy and that works for you.

When is it safe to start?

This will differ for each individual, but Sarah maintains that for most women it is safe to start from 7 to 14 days after giving birth, even if you have had a C-section or have diastasis recti. The absolute key requirements though are a knowledgable instructor who can cater for a post-natal body and to exercise very gently. And by this I do not mean joining a beginner's mat Pilates class – you can only do that six weeks after giving birth, if you feel ready. You need to start very gently to reawaken your deep core and structural muscles and focus on correcting your posture.

Why Pilates?

There are very good reasons for starting this form of exercise:

* stabilise the rib cage, which is often wider or flared post-pregnancy;

* start activating the transverse muscles and pelvic floor – the sooner you start, the better;

* improve posture as your centre of gravity and sense of balance may have changed after giving birth.

(If you are interested in trying out Pilates, look at www. pilatesperformanceireland.com for more information.)

Yoga

I really feel that yoga is something everyone should try. There are so many different types and different teachers that if you don't like one, please, please try another. I'm a huge yoga fan and I have tried many different types. I still take different classes, as I like switching things up depending on how I feel. Yoga is interesting and you really get to know your body. It's a great tool for dealing with life and all the ups and downs we experience on a daily basis. It really connects your body and mind and spirit and helps to increase your strength and flexibility. It will give you more energy, generate positivity about yourself and your body and it always helps to bring you home to yourself.

Yoga has myriad benefits for the practitioner, it can:

* improve metabolism;

* help alleviate stress and anxiety;

* improve memory;

* improve posture and balance;

* help tone your body.

Weight training

The most important thing to know is that diet is hugely responsible for achieving the healthy body you want to have. However, it is also important to realise that aerobic exercise and weight training can aid and significantly improve and speed up your progress. Weight training will not lead to bulky muscle, as you might fear. It is, in fact, the secret behind every sleek Hollywood-esque physique. I avoided weight training myself because I was terrified of bulking up, but with the encouragement of my trainer, Siobhan Byrne, I soon realised how important it is and the amazing results it delivers. It helps in the fight against osteoporosis and increases your metabolism. You can begin at any age. You can go at your pace. Far from being scary, it's an excellent exercise to incorporate into your healthy life.

For those who are not members of a gym or who don't have a trainer, there are home exercises you can do with no equipment other than a chair. Squats, lunges, dips, planks and leg raises form the core of any weight-training program for women looking to get in shape and all can be replicated effectively in the home. (You can see how to do these exercises properly earlier in this chapter or on my website, www.alisoncanavan.com, or at amandabyram.com.)

Aim to do some weight-training exercises three times a week. Time is very limited as a new mum, so begin with 20-minute sessions. For squats, do three sets of 10 reps. For lunges, do three sets of 10 reps on each leg and include the plank, as described above. Your return to exercise should be steady and not extreme. Training should be undertaken in a patient and progressive manner.

If you join a gym and you start to suffer from 'gymtimidation', please ask for help because everyone starts somewhere and if you haven't been shown how to use the machinery or weights, it's actually not common sense. I remember when I first joined a gym, I felt so insecure that I was actually afraid to ask anyone for help, but it's really important that you do in order to get the best out of your time there.

Top tip Don't return to really vigorous exercise for three months after giving birth unless you are very fit, as your body needs a rest post-birth.

Alongside the specific types of exercise listed above, there are also lots of fun classes to try, such as zumba, spin, soul cycle, yin yoga, hot yoga, clubbercise, Hit training (HITT), TRX (which is very popular with new mums as its gets results quickly) and swimming, which is an amazing, all over, gentle body workout.

How to stick to your workout routine

Show up: sounds simple, but we all know how easy it is to make excuses. The hardest part is getting there but once there, you won't regret it.

Train with a friend: it's always nice to have company, especially as a new mum as being at home alone with a baby can be hard and lonely. So make your workout social as well as sweaty!

Book it: book your class or invest in a trainer and you will feel less inclined to skip it.

Make it a habit: there is so much conflicting research out there about habits, but the general consensus is that it takes at least a couple of months to form a habit. I personally feel it's really all about routine and if you enjoy it, that's half the battle.

Reward yourself: when you reach your goals, reward yourself with a luxurious hot bath, a massage, facial or whatever your favourite indulgence is!

In case you need any more convincing, here's why I feel any and all exercise is important.

* Improves your fitness.

* It's important 'me time' for mums.

* Restores muscle strength.

* Conditions your abdominal muscles.

* Boosts your energy level.

* Gets you strong to look after your new baby (and to prepare your body for possibly another baby down the road).

* Improves your mood.

* Particular exercises, like Pilates and yoga, improve posture as your centre of gravity and sense of balance may have changed after giving birth.

* Pilates also stabilises the rib cage, which is often wider or flared post-pregnancy.

* Relieves stress.

* Helps prevent and promote recovery from post-natal depression.

It's important to remember, though, that after a caesarean birth, your recovery will be very different. It's not recommended to begin intensive abdominal work until 10–12 weeks postpartum. You need to allow extra time for connective tissue (fascia) to heal and to minimise scar tissue. I think you need to play on the side of caution and don't put that type of pressure on yourself. Really, mums, please be extra patient with yourself after major surgery.

Fitness affirmations

I am a believer in affirmations – simple phrases repeated daily to keep you focused on your goals. Use these affirmations when you are struggling, need a confidence boost or just to feel good.

1. I believe in myself and I can do anything.
2. Today I'm pushing my body so that tomorrow I can push the limits in my life.
3. As my confidence goes up, my weight goes down.
4. I am beautiful, I am fit, I am healthy.
5. I deserve a healthy and fit body and today I am working towards my goal.
6. Happiness is an attitude, not a number on the scale.
7. Good food tastes great but fit feels better – combining the two gives me strength to push through.
8. I am exercising because I love myself.
9. I will succeed at creating the body I want.
10. Today I honour my body and so I'll treat it with exercise.

Are there any physical signs that I might be trying to do too much too soon?

Yes. The most obvious sign Mother Nature sends us is that too much physical activity during the first few weeks can cause your vaginal discharge, called lochia, to become redder and to flow more heavily. This is one signal to slow down and this is your warning!

Call your doctor if vaginal bleeding restarts after you thought it had stopped or if you experience any pain when you exercise. It's important to remember that pain is not normal. If you are still suffering from lower back pain or pain in the joints after giving birth, that's an indication to schedule an appointment with a Physical Therapist. And if exercise makes you feel exhausted instead of invigorated, that's also a sign that you probably need to take it a little easier. It's also best to wait until your lochia ceases before starting to swim.

So, to recap, here are the best ways to start losing weight and regain your shape after giving birth.

My top tips to start losing weight and regain your shape after giving birth.

* Get moving as soon as you can, even if it's just for short walks. You'll be getting fresh air, aerobic exercise and, more importantly, it will help ward off baby blues and post-natal depression. Exercise motivates, which in turn generates better feelings and thoughts and more energy.

* Try doing some form of weight training.

- Squats and lunges are great for toning your hips and thighs.

- When you feel up to it and you want to really start dropping those pregnancy pounds, increase your aerobic exercise to get your heart rate up. Try walking briskly, running, swimming, or biking.

- Join a local mum and baby exercise group.

- Try yoga or Pilates as they both help to lengthen and strengthen.

- Keep modifying your choice of activity to suit how you are feeling both inside and out.

- Amanda Byram (www.amandabyram.com) has incredible fifteen-minute workouts on YouTube. She is my fitspiration queen and you will love her energy. Some of my own simple short videos with my trainer, Siobhan from Body Byrne, are also up on my site: www.alisoncanavan.com.

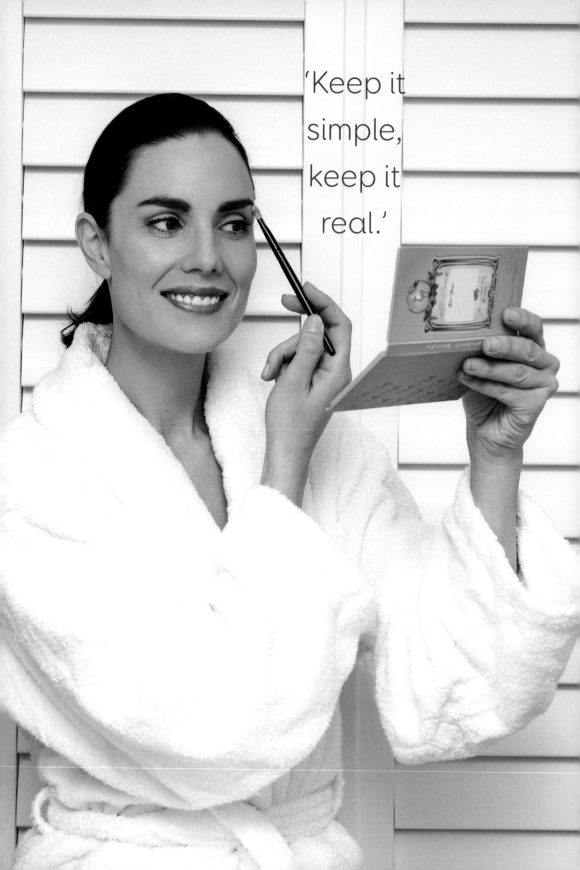

'Keep it simple, keep it real.'

BEAUTY TIPS
FOR BUSY MUMS

I f you're a new mum, you'll probably fall off the chair laughing at the memory of your pre-baby beauty and make-up routines. Suddenly your life has spun into fast-forward and you are probably wondering what shortcuts you can take. In this chapter I'm going to share with you some tips I have picked up during my 22 years as a model. There are certainly some shortcuts you can take, but the main message is to keep it simple!

Over the years there have been thousands of products applied to my face and body, but as I get older and more health-conscious I'm becoming increasingly aware of what I put on my body as well as in my body. Our skin is our largest organ and absorbs many of the chemicals in our skincare products into our blood stream. I only use natural deodorants now and I use coconut oil for pretty much everything: I use it on my body, in my hair, to take off mascara, I add it to my coffee and smoothies and I do coconut oil pulling. (For all those thinking, *What the hell?*, coconut oil pulling is an ancient ayurvedic dental technique when you swish a tablespoon of oil around in your mouth first thing in the morning to help maintain a healthy mouth. The oil has antibacterial properties and this helps to draw toxins from the body and keep teeth and gums healthy.) There are so many chemicals in all of our products now and I understand it's hard to avoid all chemicals, but we should certainly be making an effort to cut down on the amount of chemicals we are exposing ourselves to.

1.

Make-up should make you feel like a better version of you, not a different person.

This is really important because less really is more. You need to highlight your best features and not hide behind make-up. People should still be able to see the real you, just enhanced a little bit. Too much make-up makes you look older and we don't need that as tired mums! Heavy foundation and concealers often sink into fine lines and wrinkles and can look very cakey. As a young model I went to castings in New York, Paris or London with very little make-up on because the client needed to see the real me.

So think about what your favourite feature is and start from there. Do you love your eyes, eyebrows, cheeks, lips, cheekbones, skin or even your smile? Identify it, highlight it and work with it. **Don't do everything, choose what's going to be the star of the show.**

My top make-up tips for new mums

* You need to match the colour of your foundation to your skin tone and blend with your neck, as there is nothing worse than an orange face and a white neck.

* Personally, I prefer liquid concealers for under my eyes and not sticks, as sticks tend to highlight my lines. I find powders and creams can look cakey and sink into fine lines. Lightweight powders and light-reflective concealers are great alternatives.

* Use foundation that suits your skin type as a base and then cover blemishes/spots with a concealer instead of trying to apply a thick layer of foundation.

* A good natural powder foundation is also great for your handbag as it makes it quick and easy for touch-ups throughout the day. (I'd recommend Bellepierre or Bare minerals, Couleur Caramel.)

* Great eyebrows will give shape and structure to a tired face and done well they can lift your face and open your eyes. This is one shortcut all mums should take. Having your eyebrows done professionally is one less thing to worry about every day. You should only need to do this once a month, or twice if your eyebrows grow fast, but in between visits you should be able to tweeze them and keep them groomed yourself.

Prices range from €15 to €35, depending on where you go. Personally, I love Benefit Boutique for brows.

* Colour those cheeks! I always think blusher is one of the most underrated products because it can give life to your face. Too much blusher, on the other hand, can be a disaster, so go easy with it and be sure to pick a tone to suit your skin. Go lighter in summer and slightly warmer in winter and use a good blusher brush, too. Use light brush strokes so you can build up, as it's easier to add than to take away.

* I'm not a huge fan of heavy contouring and I believe it should be left in the studio or theatre, where it belongs. It doesn't translate very well in everyday life and can end up looking heavy, and make-up tends to separate on most girls. Embrace 'nontouring' as it's not normal to wear layers and layers of various shades of make-up.

* I'm a huge fan of BB (beauty balms), CC (colour correctors) and now DD (daily defence) creams as they do a multitude of things in one go and are great for busy mums on the run. They hydrate, cover, illuminate and protect the skin in one simple step.

* Wash your make-up brushes weekly. (I use Dr Bronner's soap, which can be used for pretty much anything and it's natural, too.)

My school run look or five-minute fix for hectic mornings

* Cleanse well.

* Splash cold water on your face – it wakes you up and tightens pores.

* Use a tinted moisturiser/BB/CC or DD cream.

* Then do your cheeks and apply a great blush.

* Your brows (if you get them done professionally, this step is done) – just use some powder shadow (as close as possible to your brow colour) to fill them in and brush them with a brow gel. I never use pencil as I find it looks too harsh for me, but that's a personal choice.

* Apply under-eye concealer.

* A coat of mascara on your lashes.

* Lip gloss or tinted lip balm.

> *Five minutes on my face helps boost my confidence and pace.*

As a new mum it's tempting to stay in a tracksuit all day (guilty as charged!) and not put any effort into ourselves, especially if we are at home all day. But there is no denying that when I spend even five minutes on myself, I feel better. So my new rule is five minutes on my face helps to boost my confidence and pace.

This means that if you start your day the right way, you are much more productive and you feel much better about yourself. As a mum you need to start using your time wisely – yes, you have less time to spend on yourself, but you can still feel good and look great. I like to call it minimal maintenance. I find my motivation wanes when I'm at home for a few days and make no effort to groom myself, so the key is to have a daily routine that you stick to even when the kids are hanging out of your legs.

For hair, I keep it very simple. Get a haircut that is easy to maintain and style. My hair spends most of its life in a ponytail, but a nice bun or braid are also good. To achieve a simple wavy look for long hair, braid your hair at night and shake it out in the morning and you are ready to go. Embrace natural curls. With my straight hair, I'm a fan of heated rollers, which are quick and easy to use. Layers are great for longer hair, to add texture and movement, while bobs are versatile and easy to manage. The trick is to make your hair work for you so you don't have to work hard on your hair!

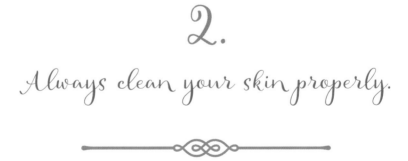

2.

Always clean your skin properly.

I have worked with some of the most successful and best make-up artists in the world and one of the things they will always do before applying your make-up is clean your skin properly.

Thoroughly cleansing the face morning and night and regular exfoliation is really important. In my opinion, it is one of the key factors in having and maintaining great skin.

Not only do you need to clean off your make-up, but also the pollutants and toxins in the air that you've picked up during the day, especially if you live in a city environment. When I first moved to London my skin took quite a while to adjust and I was shocked at how dirty my skin was at night. It was the same in New York when I was riding the subways all the time. So be diligent about cleansing thoroughly with a good cleanser, morning and night, and exfoliate dead skin cells at least once a week to help freshen your complexion. Out with the old cells and in with the new.

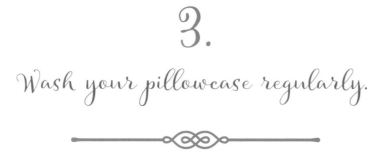

3.

Wash your pillowcase regularly.

I suffered from adult acne in my twenties and it hit again during part of my pregnancy, especially around my cheeks and chin and back of my neck and chest. If you don't change your pillowcase regularly, oil and dirt build up from your hair and skin and it keeps getting transferred back to your face, which is a very unpleasant thought.

To prevent this from happening and to help keep your skin healthy at night, follow my rule:

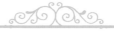

sleep – turn – sleep – wash.

So you **sleep** on one side,
then **turn** it over the following night and
sleep on the opposite side, and then **wash** it.
It's simple and effective.

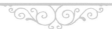

My sister Laura also swears by silk pillows as she has had sensitive skin and has suffered from eczema for years. Silk is the strongest of the natural fibres and is beneficial for skin conditions like eczema because it is incredibly smooth and soft, breathable and a natural temperature regulator. Silk contains natural cellular albumen, which speeds up the metabolism of skin cells, which in turn can help to delay the aging process. Silk is hypoallergenic and it does not attract dust mites and is a natural fungal repellent. (Check out www.theethicalsilkco.com for more information.)

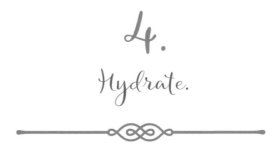

4.
Hydrate.

Radiant natural beauty comes from healthy nourished cells and the most important part of this is hydration. Drink at least six to eight glasses of water a day to help your skin stay healthy from the inside out. You can also eat your water with lots of water-rich fruits and veggies (see Chapter 5).

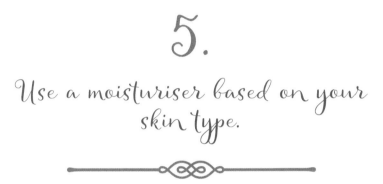

5.

Use a moisturiser based on your skin type.

The beauty industry is by far the most confusing industry on the planet, with a huge volume of information, much of it conflicting, so these days I keep it as simple as possible. One thing that is really important to use, however, is a moisturiser based on your skin type. For years I used anything that was lying around – we all think we are bulletproof in our youth! I soon learned the hard way as my skin reacted and had breakouts. It was either too clogged or dehydrated. Finding a balance is the key and getting to know your skin is essential.

When deciding on your skincare products and regime, you need to take into account the type of climate you live in and the time of year. Most of us should use lighter creams during the summer months and more nourishing creams during cold and dry weather.

How to choose the right moisturiser

So you need the right product for your skin, but how do you know your skin type? Here's how:

First and foremost, I would go to a good beautician or dermatologist to get advice and confirm your skin type, which will make it easier when you are asking for products. Once you know your skin type, the sales person in the beauty hall or pharmacy will be better able to point you in the right direction.

Combination skin: keep it simple and light so you can use it on your T-zone too. You will need a lotion to soothe dry patches without being too greasy.

Oily skin: instead of creams, look for lotions that are lightweight and non-greasy.

Dry skin: look more towards creams. I switch to creams in the winter as my skin gets dry from the heating at home. Although having said that, I do find that plant oils are amazing year-round and I use coconut oil for everything!

Normal skin: you're the lucky ones, but you still need to find a good moisturiser to keep your skin balanced. You don't need to use much, however, just apply a very thin layer.

Sensitive skin: if your skin has a tendency to completely freak out on you, look towards more natural-based products with no harsh ingredients or triggers like acids. Avoid ingredients such as Benzoyl peroxide, artificial fragrances, colourings or alcohols, Retinoids or Glycolic acid. (Not all alcohols are bad – stearyl alcohol and cetearyl alcohol are natural and safe. More info on my website!) To keep it as natural as possible, look to products from PHYTs, Kinvara, Human and Kind, Trilogy, Suki or Holos.

Using too much or too little moisturiser is not ideal. You need to try to strike a balance. I picked up the ladybird technique from the lovely people at Avene, whereby you dot the cream all over your body and then rub it in. It should sink in quickly and not feel too greasy. I use a chickpea-sized amount for my face!

Always get testers to try at home first. It's important to remember when you're making a choice that everyone is different and I would always recommend taking a sample and trying it at home before you buy anything. This is particularly important if it's an expensive product.

Top tip

Plant oils in skincare

I adore plant oils as they are easily absorbed and are packed with powerful antioxidant and anti-inflammatory compounds that nourish, protect and rejuvenate your skin. They are also similar to the kind of oil that your skin produces naturally so, just like natural foods, your body recognises them and absorbs them easily, which means your pores won't get clogged. Plant oils have also been shown to bind moisture to the skin while strengthening skin cell membranes.

When purchasing plant oils, look for natural brands. The good news is that there are plenty to choose from! Natural brands include Kinvara, Physicians Formula, Couleur Caramel, Bellepierre, Origins, Ilia, Dr Hauscka, Trilogy, Cowshed, Neals Yard, Burt's Bees, Weleda, Naif, Lavera, Barefoot SOS, Mama Mio, Suki, Jason, Human and Kind, www.greenpeople.ie, Phyt's, Biofreshskincare. ie, Natura, Holoa and naturalskincare.ie. (Another good tip:

the Kinvara face oil is amazing at removing make-up: www. kinvaraskincare.com.)

I use the majority of the following oils in place of my regular moisturiser, especially on my body. Most can be found in your local health store, or check online for stockists near you.

* **Coconut oil:** I use a raw, organic, virgin coconut oil called Coconova for cooking, frying, smoothies, make-up removal (I rub it together in my hands, apply to my face, then I use a hot facecloth to remove it) and as a body moisturiser. You can buy fractionated coconut oil (see www.alisoncanavan.com), which is liquid form, and I use this in combination with my essential oils.

* **Extra-virgin olive oil:** I use this for cooking (salads), baby's skin, my own skin. When I had long hair, swishing right down my back, I used to put olive oil on my hair, put a shower cap on and sleep in it and then shampoo it out the next morning (Dr Bronner's gets it out). My hair was incredibly shiny when I did this. Be careful not to overdo it, though, as it can end up really greasy, but my old pal apple cider vinegar (diluted) works to wash it out too.

* **Rosehip oil:** Trilogy certified rosehip oil is great. I used it during my pregnancy, on my face and belly.

* **Jojoba oil:** great for your body and for make-up removal and has also been shown to help acne sufferers because of its antibacterial and anti-inflammatory properties.

* **Aloe vera:** good quality aloe vera can be taken as a drink. It is considered a medicinal plant and has been shown to help with so many ailments, including digestive issues, immunity and reducing inflammation. You can apply it topically to burns too and it's great for canker sores and cold sores, which I can suffer from at times.

* **Shea butter:** amazing for sunburns, blemishes, skin cracks, eczema, dermatitis, cold weather and much more. Make sure you get a good quality shea butter, though, and not one that's heavily perfumed. It's the vitamin A in the shea butter that improves many conditions. If you are looking for a more nourishing moisturiser, this is for you. (I can recommend Burt's Bees shea butter as a good one.)

* **Sweet almond oil:** I like the one made by Atlantic Aromatics, which I use for my body and also put on my scalp as an anti-dandruff treatment.

* **Avocado oil:** I have a bit of a love obsession with avocado and its getting close to coconut oil for me in terms of the level of my passion for it. As well as eating them for their delicious good fats, you can use the oil for your body and hair. A friend recently told me to start putting a really good quality avocado oil on my crow's feet. This is also another great one for your post-baby belly.

You can make your own body scrubs using brown sugar and oils like coconut, sunflower, olive or indeed jojoba or sweet almond oil. I use around 1 small cup of brown sugar (I also get different-sized brown sugar crystals because, for example, bigger crystals give you a better scrub on the hip area) mixed with between ¼ to ½ cup of oil. It depends how you like it – if you want it thicker, use less oil. I also add my essential oils to everything. For a nice bedtime ritual, after a bath add lavender drops to any of your oils. Simple, quick and effective!

I'm no expert in this field, but I just love experimenting and finding things out for myself. That's the way to approach it, I think: have fun and experiment and find out what suits you best. (There's lots more below on essential oils and how to enjoy them.) Go wild with it, but do remember to stick to simple oils for your face, such as rosehip.

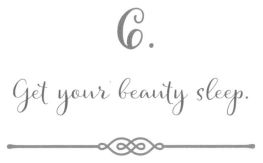

6.

Get your beauty sleep.

When you have a baby, you really start to appreciate sleep and every hour becomes precious. I presumed all my years of clubbing would stand to me, but being sober, older and staying up is just not the same. In the early days, in particular, you can feel like a zombie, so it's important to remember to rest whenever you get a chance. I know this can be hard, especially in the first few weeks, but there will come a day when you will be able to sleep again and even when you can't, some of these tips might help you to make the most of what you are getting.

Very simply, sleep is essential for your health and wellbeing and during those hours that you are in the land of nod there is magic taking place all over your body. Your cells are being renewed and rebuilt, which is vital work for your physical and mental health. Sleep is as important as food, oxygen and water.

What can you do if you struggle to sleep?

* Remove all caffeine from lunchtime onwards, and that includes all caffeinated products like tea, cola and chocolate!

* If you can, aim for a regular bedtime and try to wake up at the same time every day. As a new mum this will be hard, though; James didn't sleep through properly until he was two!

* Get that body moving every day, even if it's just a walk.

* I used to be the queen of napping but I have replaced that with meditation and I feel it's far more beneficial (see Chapter 8).

* Where you sleep is important, so make sure your bedroom is not cluttered and stuffy. There's nothing nicer than a fresh and airy room.

* Put down the gadgets at least an hour before bedtime. I did this and it helped enormously.

* Have a relaxing bedtime routine. I do some soft stretching, deep breathing and I practice gratitude (see Chapter 10) every night. I also love having a warm bath.

Another good method to try is essential oils. Personally, I love these and use them for everything – to help me focus, for calming, to aid digestion and much more. If you'd like to try this, it's important to talk to someone who is knowledgeable about oils. (You can contact Caroline at www.honestabouthealth.com or me at www.alisoncanavan.com.) When selecting essential oils, you need to choose 100% pure oils for the safest and most effective health benefits. Essential oils can be used aromatically to affect mood and open airways; topically for quick absorption into the body through the skin; and internally for immune and digestive support.

Top four essential oils for sleep

1. **Lavender**
   It's widely known that lavender promotes emotional balance and is commonly used for sleep issues. Before bed, apply lavender topically to the soles of the feet or diffuse in a room.

2. **Vetiver**
   Vetiver is a natural tranquiliser and for that reason

is known as the 'oil of tranquility'. If suffering from insomnia, apply this oil to the bottoms of your feet or to the spine. Diffuse vetiver in the bedroom at night to aid a restful night's sleep.

3. **Majoram**

Majoram blends well with lavender and is another great oil for emotional balance. It has a calming effect and helps ease feelings of anxiety. If feeling stressed about sleeping, apply majoram to the back of the neck and soles of the feet before bed.

4. **Roman chamomile**

Roman chamomile is often used for overexcitement, which makes it a popular choice for parents of boisterous children. Diffusing at night promotes emotional balance and helps with insomnia.

Tart Montmorency cherries are amazing to help you sleep. I drink a concentrated cherry drink every night (Apothecherry or Cherry Active). It has lots of melatonin to encourage a restful sleep and I find it also helps me to relax. It's a potent antioxidant and anti-inflammatory too, which is great as it also helps fight aging. A good all-rounder then! Sold!

Top tip

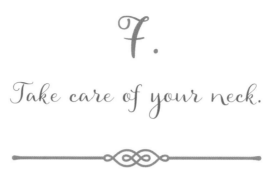

7.

Take care of your neck.

———————⚬⚭⚬———————

This is a crucial piece of advice: take care of your neck! It's the one place we neglect, but one of the first places to show our age. (I read Nora Ephron's wonderful book *I Feel Bad About My Neck* recently, and in it she describes how a plastic surgeon told her that 43 is a watershed year for necks! According to her source, the skin on the neck starts to lose elasticity when we hit 43, which is a very sobering thought.) So many of us moisturise our body and our face and then completely forget about our neck. If you want to give it a chance of remaining youthful, moisturise your neck morning and night.

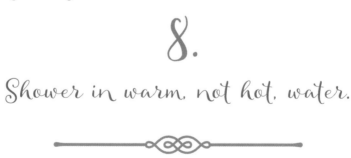

8.

Shower in warm, not hot, water.

———————⚬⚭⚬———————

I like to shower in warm water as hot water dehydrates the skin and causes premature aging. I always apply my moisturiser straight after too, while my skin is still damp.

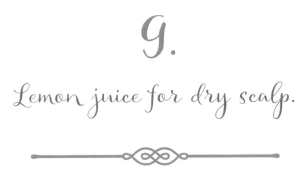

9.

Lemon juice for dry scalp.

⸻⸺⟨⟨⟩⟩⸻⸺

I suffer from dry scalp from time to time and a hairdresser in NYC once told me to squeeze lemon juice onto my scalp as the acidity exfoliates your scalp and clears the dandruff. I had terrible dry scalp after James was born and this homebrew really worked. The added bonus is that it's natural and inexpensive.

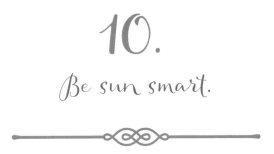

10.

Be sun smart.

⸻⸺⟨⟨⟩⟩⸻⸺

You might notice that I didn't just say 'use sunscreen' here and that's because there's more to being sun smart than just slapping on cream. I spent time in Australia modelling and I adored it, but I also love their motto for their sun smart campaign: Slip, Slap, Slop, Seek, Slide. In other words, slip on a long-sleeved shirt, slap on a hat, slop on sunscreen, seek shade and slide on your sunnies.

Only one-fifth of that excellent advice concerns sunscreen and that's because being sun smart also requires you to:

* stay out of the midday sun;

* dress appropriately and wear breathable fabrics and also don a hat and sunglasses;

* stay in the shade when you can;

* use sunscreen in both the winter and summer months. Contrary to popular belief, the winter sun is just as damaging so wearing an SPF all year round is key.

Pregnancy-related beauty issues

Chloasma

Chloasma (or the Mask of Pregnancy) refers to splashes of darkened skin that may appear on the forehead, nose and cheeks in a mask-like configuration on some pregnant women, more often in dark-skinned women. These changes may be triggered by hormonal changes during pregnancy and by the sun. I developed it on my face after a holiday in Spain. I had pigmented patches on my forehead and around my mouth. The areas of increased pigmentation will probably fade within a few months after delivery (as mine did) and your skin should return to its normal shade.

I probably sat out for too long on that occasion and in the future I would avoid the sun altogether if I was to become pregnant again. The effects of the sun on chloasma are not to be underestimated as doctors believe that even strong indoor lights can trigger and exacerbate the condition. Post-pregnancy there are many treatments available to target this problem. For example, around six months after I had James I went to a dermatologist and had a skin peel, which was successful.

Post-pregnancy there are over-the-counter products that you can ask your pharmacist for, but be patient and give it time. I became quite clever with make-up to disguise it, using darker/lighter powders on the areas that were pigmented. I also used concealer and bronzer to great effect. I will admit this level of deception does take practice, though!

SkinCeuticals Pigment Regulator is a very good product. It's proven to be effective on brown spots, freckles, dark patches and blotchiness and helps prevent future discolourations without unhealthy side-effects. The NeoStrata Pigment Lightening Gel is also highly effective against the unattractive pigmentation that affects up to 50% of expectant mums. It can be used to treat the face, chest, shoulders and hands. (*Note: it is advised to consult your physician before using the gel if breast-feeding.*)

Sometimes, the chloasma extends into deeper layers of the skin and can 'settle in'. Your dermatologist may recommend a stronger skin cream, bleach or a chemical peel, dermabrasion, or even laser treatment.

- **A chemical peel** entails a solution being applied to the skin, which causes it to peel off over a few days. New skin grows in to replace the blistered areas.

- **Dermabrasion** will remove the surface skin cells with a rapidly rotating brush. This procedure will leave skin red and sensitive and you will need to stay out of the sun for a few months.

Laser treatment uses a narrow laser beam to target skin cells. (There can be many side-effects with this treatment, so ask your beautician and talk it through fully first.)

Always know that there are options available to treat such problems but that prevention is the best route, of course, so wear a high SPF all year round. This is really important, and especially during pregnancy. The key here is to look for paraben-free sunscreens. Parabens and toxins contained in everyday beauty products have been linked to cancer and other diseases, so it really is time we educated ourselves and chose better options with regard to our sunscreens, deodorants and shampoos.

How can you tell what the better options are? Well, thankfully there is a fantastic website, www.ewg.org, which has the most comprehensive and up-to-date advice and research, along with a list of approved products, so just log on and download a list of safe products. Alternatively, search your favourite products to see if they are safe, it's that simple. The aim of the Environmental Working Group (EWG) is to empower people to live healthier lives in a healthier environment using breakthrough research and education.

Stretch marks

Stretch marks come in all shapes and sizes. I was very lucky to escape with none on my belly, but not so lucky around my hips and thighs. My hips was where I put on weight first, and fast, and when I lost it I ended up with quite a lot of stretch marks there. At least half of pregnant women get stretch marks and research suggests that your genetics play a big role in whether you will develop them or not. If your mum or sister had them after birth, your chances of developing them are much higher.

The most common area that stretch marks develop is the belly as it expands rapidly to accommodate your growing baby. Some mums will get them on their buttocks, thighs, hips and breasts. Stretch marks are caused by changes in the elastic supportive tissue that lies just beneath the skin. They start out pink, reddish brown, purple or dark brown, depending on your skin colour.

You'll be happy to hear that stretch marks do fade, but I'm afraid they never disappear totally. I find that consistent moisturising is essential to help prevent and treat them. Coconut oil is great and can also be used on C-section scars. I like to call them 'love lines' – at least that's what I told James when he asked me what the wrinkly things were when he saw me in my bikini on holidays! If I have to live with them, then I'm going to think of them as souvenirs of creating my little man who makes me smile every day, then it seems a small price to pay.

Top tips on how to handle stretch marks

* I used coconut oil throughout my pregnancy and found it particularly good for the itching I experienced. My belly used to itch like crazy, especially towards the end, and I remember getting funny looks when I was out as I would scratch without thinking!

* I would also add some coconut oil to my bath in the evenings to make it extra moisturising. (WARNING: be very careful as it can make it slippy, so use a non-slip bathmat for safety.)

* Moisturise twice a day: morning and night.

* Drink six to eight glasses of water a day, eat healthily and exercise.

* Stretch marks will fade over time, but if you are particularly worried, contact a dermatologist and he/she will be able to advise on specialist treatments.

Pregnancy and post-pregnancy acne

As noted earlier, I suffered from adult acne both before and after I had James. Funnily enough, it cleared up completely during the last trimester of my pregnancy. Again, the acne is down to your hormones and often occurs during the first trimester, usually appearing around the chin and jaw area. Some mums may experience breakouts on their neck and back, too. If you suffer, you are not alone – more than one out of every two women can be affected by it. Stress can also be a contributing factor, which will be discussed in full in Chapter 9.

Giving birth can also trigger post-pregnancy acne, so be careful with your treatment decisions if you are breastfeeding and avoid products containing acne-fighting ingredients like salicylic acid and benzoyl peroxide until you've finished breastfeeding. Give your body time to regulate its hormone levels, which takes longer when you are feeding, and focus on a good skincare routine.

I have taken many different medications for my acne and they worked temporarily, but since I have cleaned up my lifestyle and diet and limited my dairy intake, my skin is much better. You need to figure out what works for you, but try everything and not just one thing so, for example, good eating habits, sleep, positive mental attitude and a good skincare regime combined will help. If it persists, consult your dermatologist.

There is an amazing product from biofresh skincare (www.biofreshskincare.ie) called Acne Out and it kills the bacteria immediately and the spots disappear.

Varicose veins

Varicose veins are caused by a combination of factors during pregnancy. They can also be hereditary; my grandmother, Mum and sister all developed them. Your body has more of the hormone progesterone during pregnancy, which relaxes your blood vessel walls, and the extra weight gain from your growing baby bump puts significant pressure on the veins trying to carry blood back to your heart.

Veins have valves, which stop the blood that is returning to your heart from flowing backwards. Varicose veins develop when the valves don't work properly, and the vein walls become weak, enlarged and twisted due to the backpressure and they appear close to the surface of the skin. When this happens, you can experience pain, throbbing, aching, tiredness, heaviness, cramps, burning, itching, restless legs and swelling. They can also cause blood clots and lead to more serious conditions, such as bleeding veins and leg ulcers.

It's completely understandable if you want to do something about them and bare your pins again, especially during the summer months. There are treatments available, including a new revolutionary treatment called The Venaseal Closure System (www.venaseal.com). This treatment requires only a local anaesthetic and promises immediate results.

How you can prevent/minimise varicose veins during pregnancy:

* get some exercise daily – even a 10-minute walk will help boost circulation;

* elevate your feet and legs whenever possible. Use a stool or box to rest your legs on when you're sitting, and keep your feet elevated on a pillow when you're lying down;

* don't sit or stand for long periods;

* eat healthily and try to keep within the recommended weight range for each stage of pregnancy;

* wear support stockings all day, especially in the latter stages of pregnancy – they are available in most pharmacies;

* your large vein, the inferior cava, is on the right side so sleep on your left side, which will relieve the vein from the weight of your uterus;

* sometimes they are simply hereditary, so contact your GP if they are painful and bothering you.

Hair loss post-pregnancy

What new mum doesn't get a fright when clumps of her hair start to clog the shower drain? But don't panic and be assured that this is all completely normal. I had clumps of hair around my forehead fall out and I was stuck with baby hair for quite a while, which looked a little odd.

During your pregnancy you might have the hair you've always dreamed of: thick, shiny and lustrous! But those inevitable hormonal changes lead to increased estrogen in the body during pregnancy, which causes your hair to stay in what's called a 'resting phase' for longer. Post-pregnancy, when your estrogen drops, you lose the hair that you would normally lose daily plus all the extra hair that you have not lost during your pregnancy, so please don't panic.

How to manage your post-pregnancy hair:

* use a volume-boosting shampoo;

- use shampoos and conditioners for thin hair as they won't weigh down your hair so much;

- get a new haircut to make your hair look fuller and it will also be easier to manage;

- don't use tight elastic to tie back your hair;

- use hairbands and accessories – on holidays, when I was very paranoid, I used nice headscarfs and bandanas beside the pool and pretty hairbands in the evening;

- just remember that this too shall pass and easy does it, so go very gently with your hair to minimise large losses in one go;

- I used to brush through every morning with my natural bristle paddle brush to avoid large amounts falling out as I went about my day;

- no tight towels on your head after showering or bathing as they pull the hair too much.

Serums and eye creams

Serums

I was a serum virgin until a few years ago as I really didn't understand what they were for, or indeed if they were any use. I now use them religiously as a preventative and corrective measure. Serums are light, fast-absorbing liquids used as an alternative or in addition to creams or lotions. The biggest difference between a serum and a cream or lotion is what the formulation doesn't include. Serums leave out occlusive, or airtight, moisturising ingredients, such as petrolatum, a mineral oil jelly that prevents water from evaporating. They also contain fewer lubricating and thickening agents, like nut or seed oils. Most serums are water-based, eliminating oils altogether.

As you're left with such a high concentration of active ingredients with a serum, most dermatologists would recommend them. They can have powerful antioxidants in them and are great to have on your team in the fight against aging. Serums can be the costliest part of your skincare range because of the ingredients used, but you only need a tiny amount for each application, which means it should last for quite a while. They are made of very small molecules, so the skin absorbs them quickly and deeply. Thicker creams, on the other hand, form a barrier on your skin, which is great for locking in moisture but can also lock active ingredients out.

> " *Our skin is a reflection of what's going on inside our body. With a few small tweaks to your diet and lifestyle, turning back the hands of time may not be such a huge feat after all.* "

The main function of a serum is to help correct damage from the past and protect from future damage at a deeper level. They can be used on sensitive skin, too, but bear in mind that serums aren't for everyone. The liquid or gel-like texture of a serum can be a poor match for people with chronic skin conditions like eczema or rosacea, which weaken the skin barrier. For these people, serums may penetrate too quickly, causing irritation.

Eye creams

We all have different skin types, lifestyles and needs, so it stands to reason that in the area of eye creams, or indeed gels, we're all looking for something different. But what works and what's the difference between the two?

There is a huge difference between the two primarily because eye creams hydrate throughout the day and evening, while eye gels are meant to be more sheer, therefore penetrating into the skin and enabling more corrective work, for example puffiness, fine lines and dark circles.

As eye gels are lighter weight, younger people usually favour them. Eye gels are more soothing and cooling for tired eyes and ideal for reducing puffiness because the main way you reduce puffiness is by soothing and cooling the area around the eye. Eye gels are also absorbed much faster so they're great for busy women on the go as they leave little residue and you can apply your make-up quickly. Rose water is great as it's a natural anti-inflammatory, or cucumber!

Trilogy Age Proof CoQ10 Eye Recovery Concentrate, which is available in pharmacies, is the perfect pick-me-up for tired eyes as the gently massaging roll-on applicator helps to stimulate circulation, while carefully selected lightening, brightening and tightening actives work their age-proofing wonders. This one is a great handbag essential as it can be used over make-up, instantly reviving you any time, day or night.

Eye creams, on the other hand, are far more nourishing and moisturising. Creams contain more ingredients that moisturise the skin more effectively than gels. Most experts will tell you to use a cream for mature skin, as you need more oil to improve its health. Creams eventually leave aging skin with fine lines looking much better than before because they contain emollients that nourish the skin and plump up the area, helping to eliminate those fine lines. They are also better for people who suffer from dry skin.

Whatever your skin needs, there's an eye gel or cream for you that will help prevent those inevitable wrinkles. With our busy lives these days, we need all the help we can get!

Dental care post-pregnancy

During your pregnancy you might notice your gums becoming tender. It's advisable to go for a full check-up to take care of your dental health once the baby is born. Regular periodontal (gum) exams are very important because pregnancy causes hormonal changes that put you at increased risk for periodontal disease and for tender gums that bleed easily – a condition called pregnancy gingivitis. Pay particular attention to any changes in your gums during pregnancy. If tenderness, bleeding or gum swelling occurs at any time during your pregnancy, talk with your dentist or periodontist as soon as possible. And of course, you must follow really good oral hygiene practices to prevent and/or reduce oral health problems, so brush, floss and rinse! I received great post-natal care from www.mydental.ie, who have been looking after my teeth and gums since I had James. They also look after your children for free if you are a patient!

Final thought

So even though your new arrival, or (if you're like my friend Caroline – four kids under 2½!!) arrivals are demanding and adorable, you still need to continue with some kind of beauty routine. Yes, you have to pare it down, but you can still have fun. Remember that taking care of yourself in this way is important – it's self-care, relationship-care and future-proofing rolled into one!

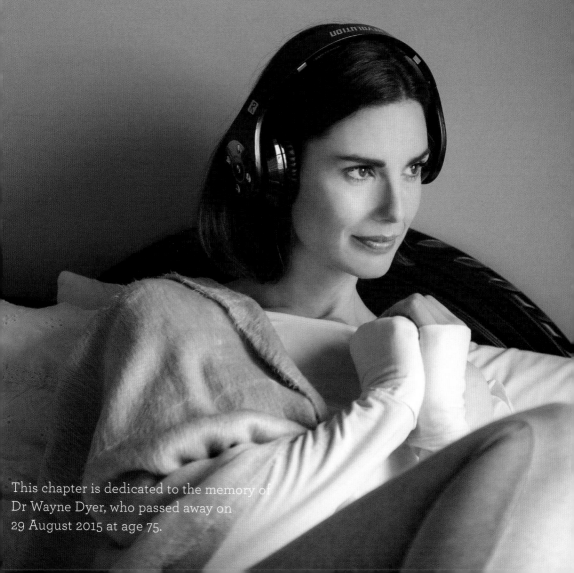

'Develop an appreciation for the present moment. Seize every second of your life and savour it.'
Dr Wayne Dyer

This chapter is dedicated to the memory of Dr Wayne Dyer, who passed away on 29 August 2015 at age 75.

8

MINDFULNESS AND MEDITATION

I do believe mindfulness and meditation are essential for everyone and I don't write that sentence lightly. I dipped in and out of meditation throughout my early career in London in the mid- to late 1990s when I first took up yoga. At the beginning of every class we would set our intentions and at the end of the practice we said 'Thank you' and did some meditation, and I have never looked back! I have been meditating for many years, but it was really during my time in New York (2003–2010) that I explored this whole area a lot deeper. There are many different types of meditation and I have practiced quite a few in my time. I now practice primordial sound meditation on a daily basis, but sometimes I use guided meditation and I also use music, depending on my mood. Throughout the years I have developed my own meditations that help me with day-to-day life, which I will share with you at the end of the chapter.

Whilst a certain type of meditation might not work for everyone, it is essential that we all slow down and at least try to spend some time in the present moment every day. To me, meditation, mindfulness or 'mindfulness meditation' all mean the same thing, which is very simply just being in the moment.

As I learned at The Chopra Institute, meditation is a journey from activity into silence. It helps us on our journey towards inner peace and releases stress and tension.

> ## This is How I See It:
> ## Meditation: Go Within
> ## Mindfulness: Live in the Moment

Mindfulness is all about being in the moment. For example, when you are talking to someone, actually talk to them and be wholly present. For me it's really about paying attention to what is happening right now.

Meditation: the busier you are, the more you need it

We live in crazy times where we rarely get to catch our breath and sit still. My spiritual journey has been wonderful, scary and hilarious at times. I've had meditation teachers who told me to clear my brain of all thoughts (not possible, by the way), but then I had teachers like Kadem Mortem (Kadampa Buddhism) in New York City who has an incredible capacity to speak to New Yorkers in a language they understand. After his meditations and lessons I always seemed to be able to make sense of my life there. Through him I learned how to be more compassionate with both others and myself. In fact, it was during my difficult times when I returned to Ireland that I was able to recall all his lessons and teachings, which helped me to heal.

Deepak Chopra and Dr Wayne Dyer are two people who have had a huge impact on my life and journey and, of course, Oprah Winfrey because in my opinion Oprah is the magic marker that helps us to join the dots within ourselves, encouraging us to dig deep, think, believe, be and do. Dr Wayne Dyer's teachings helped me through some of the most difficult times in my life. I had just watched his movie *The Shift* for the third time the night he passed away and if you haven't seen it, you must seek it out. It's a movie that looks at how to find your purpose in life and I really feel it's the must-see movie for our generation.

The biggest addiction we have in modern society is negative thinking, and meditation can help with this. The mind really is the root of everything. It's the creator of both happiness and suffering. Buddha says that all our fear and anxiety comes from a mind that's untamed, leaving me with one thought: why not try meditation?

I know I've said it before, but it's worth repeating. You are in control, so exercise that control with my negative thought catcher:

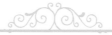

Stop – Catch – Change

Stop your thought.

Catch it (sometimes I actually use my hand for this and it really helps).

Change it to a new more positive thought about yourself, your situation or someone else!

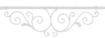

We can practice mindfulness and meditation in so many ways and by the end of this chapter I hope you will find it impossible not to practice it in some form or another. I used to put meditation on my To Do list, almost like another chore, until one day I realised it had become a part of me and was just as important as eating and sleeping. I love my daily meditation and if I don't practice, I really notice the difference. The magic of meditation does not happen during the practice but rather outside of it, in your everyday life.

> " **Stress is our biggest killer and meditation can help us to cope.** "

Here are just a few things I have noticed about myself through regular meditation practice: I sleep better, feel more content and I'm more creative. The big change for me, however, is that I can cope with stress, stressful situations, toddler tantrums, work issues, addictions/cravings, family problems and college work a lot easier. It won't solve all your problems, but it will absolutely help you to cope better with them.

As my ability to cope with daily stresses has become better, I have also found that I am much more positive and that my energy has changed. You start attracting more of what you want into your life. For me, meditation has enabled me to find my true path and live my truth.

You don't have to take my word for it, though, as these days there is lots of scientific research to back up these assertions. It has been scientifically proven, for example, that meditation can alter the structure and function of the brain, which is called **neuroplasticity** and is basically the brain's ability to change and adapt.

Meditation activates a part of the brain associated with positive emotions. Even when you are not practicing these areas are still lit up, proving that mental training does affect the brain. There have been many studies on the effects of meditation on brain structure and the findings suggest that long-term meditators have structural differences in both gray and white matter. (To read up on it for yourself, go to http://scan.oxfordjournals.org/content/8/1/27.abstract.)

> " *Meditation gives peace in a world gone mad.* "

Gray matter controls learning, memory and our sense of wellbeing, but both gray and white matter are major components of the Central Nervous System (CNS), which includes the brain and the spinal cord. The brain and spinal cord together make-up the body's main control centre, almost like a headquarters. As far as I'm concerned, it just makes sense to work at HQ and take control of what's going on in our body and mind. Go straight to the top, I say![4]

There is no right or wrong way to practice meditation and quite simply if you are doing it, you are doing it right.

Through my studies I have definitely learned how to deepen my practice, but as a busy mum just remembering to **stop, breathe and be** is all you need to do!

Stop, breathe and be.

---

4 Source: 'The Central Nervous System (CNS).' *Boundless Psychology. Boundless*, 14 Sep. 2015. Retrieved 6 Oct. 2015 from https://www.boundless.com/psychology/textbooks/boundless-psychology-textbook/biological-foundations-of-psychology-3/the-nervous-system-34/the-central-nervous-system-cns-147-12682/.

Becoming more mindful

The first step is to become more mindful of everyday things, like eating meals, playing with your kids and talking to people. Have you ever felt like you are speaking to someone and their mind is elsewhere? Few of us are ever really focused in the moment and really listening and engaged. We are either thinking about what we didn't do or errands we have to run. As a new mum you might find that you are anxious and worried about the baby and often as parents we are always thinking way too far ahead.

So please mums:

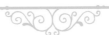

Catch – Stop – Think

Catch yourself

Stop

Think – enjoy the moment

I think everyone should include daily therapy/mindfulness in their day-to-day lives. I use the word therapy here because I don't believe that therapy is a word that just describes sitting in a specialist's room. I firmly believe that our health and wellbeing is a daily job that needs to be worked on.

Simple, everyday things like dancing and singing are examples of great therapy that we can include in our daily lives. Art is therapy, friendship is therapy, so meditation is also therapy and self-care of any kind can be counted as therapy, too. How about a bubble bath, a walk in the park, coffee with friends or enjoying a cup of tea by yourself? To me, therapy is anything that contributes to a positive and balanced lifestyle.

20 therapeutic/mindful ideas for you to try

1. Buy fresh flowers: as a single mum I started to do this and I love having fresh flowers in my house as they really brighten my day.

2. Take a bubble bath: this can be tough as a new mum; I think I have had only a handful of showers without an audience since I have become a mum! But if you do get the time, a bubble bath is a wonderful indulgence.

3. Swing: no, you didn't read it wrong. Swing on the swings in the playground and see how high you can go. This is one of my favourite things to do and now James can do it with me too!

4. Listen to music: fast or slow music feeds the soul. I often have solo discos at home alone when I want to blow off steam or just let my hair down. It makes you laugh, especially when you do it with your kids.

5. Sing your heart out: many things get lost on our transition into adulthood and singing is usually one of them, but it actually has huge benefits and is a great release. Sing your heart out, right now as you are reading this, and notice how you feel. I bet you feel better?

6. Read: read your favourite book or a book you have had your eye on for a while. You might laugh and think I am completely crazy because as a mum you simply have no time, but if reading is a passion of yours, find just 10 minutes a day to do it. Maybe when the kids have gone to sleep before you begin the evening cleaning (I know, it never ends).

7. Have a cup of tea and your favourite treat: this is one you can do with someone you love, or deliciously alone!

8. Organise a get-together with friends: girly chats always help!

9. Meditate.

10. Colour: yes, adult colouring is wonderful and I find it helps me to focus and reduces my anxiety. It's also great fun!

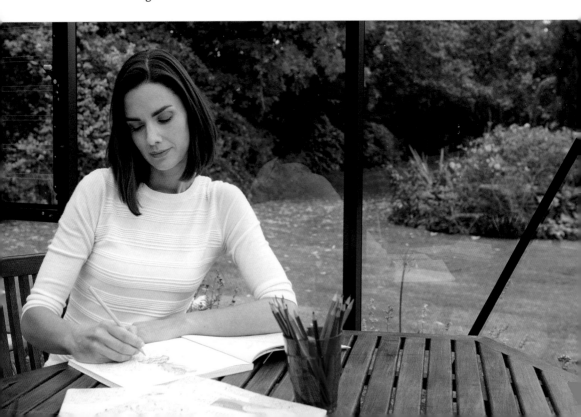

11. **Knit or sew:** both very relaxing. As the kids get older and you find yourself waiting around for dance or music classes to finish, things like knitting are a great way to pass the time and practice mindfulness.

12. **Laugh!:** laugh at yourself, a funny movie, a silly book.

13. **Go for a walk:** walking is great for everyone and clears the head and gets your circulation going. It can also boost mood and energy.

14. **Cook your favourite meal:** there is nothing nicer than sitting down to your all-time favourite meal; cooking can be relaxing and therapeutic too.

15. **Take a nap:** anytime someone offers to take the baby or mind the kids, don't even hesitate to jump into that bed for a nap. You deserve it!

16. **Journal:** write down your ideas, dreams, hopes and worries. I find writing one of the greatest forms of therapy. You don't have to be a good writer to do this.

17. **Squeeze a stress ball:** I love them as they help to release tension and stress.

18. **Try yoga or pilates:** you might just find you love it, and it will certainly help to regain your shape and keep you calm and focused.

19. **Give yourself a compliment:** that's right, every single day pay yourself a compliment.

20. **Breathing:** breathing is essential, free and acessible to us all at any time, yet it is the most underused resource we have. So check in with yourself a few times a day and just breathe – take three to five deep breaths.

As you can see from this list, being mindful is about finding something you like to do and making the time for it and enjoying it. I set alarms on my phone at intervals throughout the day to remind myself to breathe and check in with myself. I also have post-it notes on my computer with quotes and motivations! If you are struggling as a new mum, I promise you that breathing and taking time out for yourself will make a world of difference.

Meditation

I know most new mums will say they don't have the time to meditate, which is exactly why you should try it. The key is to find a practice you like and are comfortable with. If you enjoy it and look forward to it, you will have no problem fitting it into your life.

Even more than that, though, meditation actually gives me my time back because I am more focused, energetic, relaxed and clear about my intentions, which saves time in the long run. Meditation has enabled me to achieve a lot more in my life. I went from being sick, tired, overwhelmed and stressed to being energetic, calm, focused and alive! Meditation brings me back to myself and keeps me motivated.

I have practiced meditation with James present since he was a baby and I still do. At five years of age he sometimes comes and sits with me while I meditate and sometimes he doesn't. I never expect anything from him, but at least he has been introduced to the idea of just being. After all, we are human beings and not human doings! When he was a baby I used to make sure he was safe in his cot or playpen and I would meditate just for 5–10 minutes. If he's worried now, we hold hands and meditate and it's a really beautiful time together.

Meditation has also helped me to heal from a broken heart, loss of a loved one and much more. Through meditation, emotions that have been buried for a long time can surface and although this has not been easy to deal with it, it has been necessary. Buried emotions are like ticking time-bombs waiting to go off and the earlier you deal with them, the better. Mine were buried for well over 30 years so there was a good bit of work to be done, but as I have said before, it's all about joining the dots for ourselves and doing what is necessary at the time and in our own time.

Through meditation I now tune in and listen to what my body is trying to tell me. Some days I have a great meditation and some days I find it hard to sit still. The trick is not to expect fireworks, an out-of-body experience or the Lotto numbers to appear during meditation! Some people get so attached to the outcome of something miraculous happening that they can feel let down and a bit disappointed by the calm reality. To be honest, the real magic happens outside of meditation. You just have to trust the process.

Most people think you have to meditate in lotus position in front of an altar or lighted candles, but I meditate anywhere I am lucky enough to have time, which means planes, trains, in the car before a meeting, on the beach, at home, at work (during a break). That's the thing about being a mum, you will start to wonder what you used to do with all your time before.

mums + meditation = match!

The body gets a deep level of rest during meditation and as rest is what new mums are missing, it just makes sense that you need to find a match for what you are missing.

Consistent and constant practice is the key and you can start from as little as five minutes a day. Just remember, five minutes every day is better than 40 minutes at the weekend. Do you scroll through social media for five minutes a day? If so, you have the time to meditate. I learned the necessity of consistency the hard way – by not doing it. For years I used to head off on long retreats and weekend retreats or just meditate on Tuesdays and Thursdays and then leave long gaps in between my practice. It didn't work. I couldn't join the dots with my loss of connection within myself a few days later. It took me a while, but I finally cottoned on to the fact that the problem was lack of consistency.

So to help you get in touch with yourself, I am sharing three of my personal guided meditations that I use for different times of the day, or whenever I feel I need them. They are also available for you to download from my website at www.alisoncanavan.com.

Top tip

The main thing to remember during meditation is not to block your thoughts. Acknowledge them, but don't follow them. Think of it like watching traffic and then all of a sudden you see your favourite car, like a red Ferrari, and you are tempted to follow it. Don't follow, just let it go by!

Each morning I have a routine: as soon as I open my eyes I say *Thank you* as I put my feet on the ground. As I get out of the bed, I sit up and take three deep breaths and then do some simple gentle stretches (see www.alisoncanavan.com for more). Then I go and drink a large glass of lemon water and on the way I always light an incense stick and if I forget, James reminds me! So try some or all of this. It will take a while for it to become habit but when it does, you will find it helps enormously because starting your day this way means you are calm and focused. (I used to leave a post-it note on my phone saying 'breathe' as we all know that's one of the first things most of us reach for each morning – and if we have time to scroll through our phone, we have time for a few deep breaths and a stretch!)

If you have never tried meditation before, there are various different types you can try. There are lots of Apps and guided meditations around, but my advice is to keep it simple. Sit still, close your eyes and notice the natural flow of your breath. Observe your breath for a few minutes and notice the changes in how you feel. Does it help you to feel more relaxed? As a beginner you can simply start here and add a minute to your practice every few days or every week, aiming to eventually reach 20 minutes a day. This can take time; it took me well over a year to reach a full 20 minutes each day. Just do what you can.

> *Meditation is not just for yogis, monks and what we consider spiritual people – it's for everyone.*

The three meditations

#1: Protection

This meditation will help to protect you from negativity. I do this if I know I'm going to be in difficult company or around negative people. It's great if you are feeling vulnerable and if you find you pick up on people's negative energies easily. So if you tend to be exhausted after meeting certain people or if you know you are going to be in company you find challenging (in-laws, family members or work colleagues you don't get on with), then my advice is to spend 10 minutes on yourself first.

To begin:

Sit comfortably in an upright position. (For all of these meditations I advise people not to lie down, especially new mums, as they have a tendency to fall asleep and meditation is about being present.)

Relax your shoulders and inhale deeply, then exhale deeply and close your eyes.

On the next inhalation, breathe in for the count of five.

1
2
3
4
5

Hold for two seconds.

1
2

And then let it out slowly.

Repeat this five times, and then on the next inhalation imagine you are breathing in pure white light through your nose. When your breath reaches the top of your head the white light explodes gently, like a firework, and trickles down through your body. First your head, then down your neck and into your chest area. With every in breath the white light goes deeper into your body, continuing down through your abdomen, into your arms and down your legs until eventually your entire body is filled with white light from your fingertips right down to your toes.

When you have finished filling your body with light internally, I want you to visualise yourself stepping into a white light suit and zip it up from your toes to the top of your head and repeat silently to yourself three times:

I am surrounded by pure white light,

I am surrounded by pure white light,

I am surrounded by pure white light.

Continue to breathe in and out for a few minutes, enjoying your light-filled body.

In just a few moments I will count down from five to one and when I reach number one you will open your eyes, re-energised, protected and ready for the day ahead.

5

4

3

2

1

Open your eyes and thank you for a great meditation.

(If you find yourself in a difficult position at any stage throughout your day, you can ask your angels to protect you with white light by repeating three times, 'Archangel Michael, protect me now'.)

#2: Relaxation

I use lots of different visualisation meditations for myself if I'm finding it hard to relax. I adore the ocean and the beach, so here's one that always works for me and I hope it helps you too.

Sit comfortably in an upright position.

Relax your shoulders and inhale deeply and then exhale deeply and close your eyes.

On the next inhalation, breathe in for the count of five.

1
2
3
4
5

Hold for two seconds.

1
2

And then let it out slowly.

Continue to breathe like this for a few minutes.

Imagine you are all alone, walking on a white sandy beach. As you walk along you can feel the warm sun on your face and a light breeze in your hair. As you look down you notice the beautiful soft white sand in between your toes and with each step you take, the softness of the sand helps you to feel calm and safe.

You take a seat at the water's edge and listen to the soft waves as the water covers your feet and ankles and then retreats back to the sea. You watch the sea come and go for quite a while as you observe the ease of movement and the natural flow of the sea.

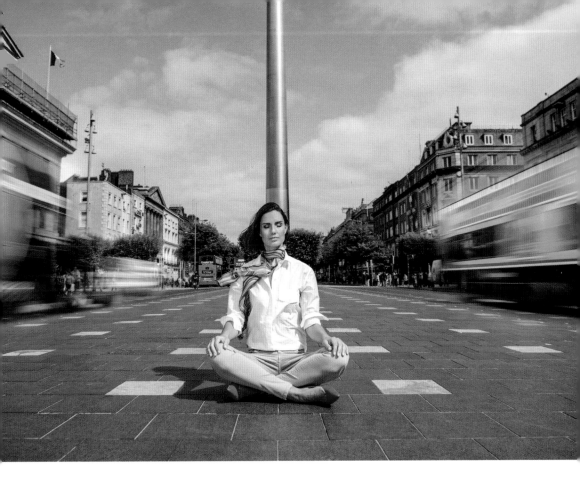

I want you to keep that feeling with you throughout your day and every time you get stressed, just think of the soft sand moving through your toes and the gentle sea washing all your troubles away.

Now I'm going to count down from five to one and when I reach number one you will open your eyes and feel refreshed, relaxed, energised and ready for your day.

5
4
3
2
1

Open your eyes and thank you for a great meditation.

#3: Dump your day

We've all been there, the day from hell – and as a mum it could well include being covered in sick, wee, milk and more. We all have those days when things go wrong and all we want to do is go to bed and wake up again. Sometimes I can find it hard to let go of things and I need to work through a letting go process, which is a combination of journaling, talking and what I call my 'dump my day' meditation. During the meditation I breathe in white light and exhale grey/black air, which symbolises my used-up energy/emotions and generally all the things I am done with for the day.

To begin:

Sit comfortably in an upright position.

Relax your shoulders and inhale deeply and then exhale deeply and close your eyes.

On the next inhalation, breathe in for the count of five.

1

2

3

4

5

Hold for two seconds.

1

2

And then let it out slowly.

Continue to breathe like this for a few minutes.

On your next in breath imagine you are breathing in fresh, pure white light and as you exhale, you are exhaling all the used-up air and energy from your day. Continue to breathe like this until you have imagined that the white light has replaced all the negative emotions of your day.

As we come to the end of the meditation I'm going to count down from five to one and when I reach number one you will open your eyes, feeling lighter and refreshed, and you will be ready for a good night's sleep in preparation for a fresh new start tomorrow.

5
4
3
2
1

Open your eyes and thank you for a great meditation.

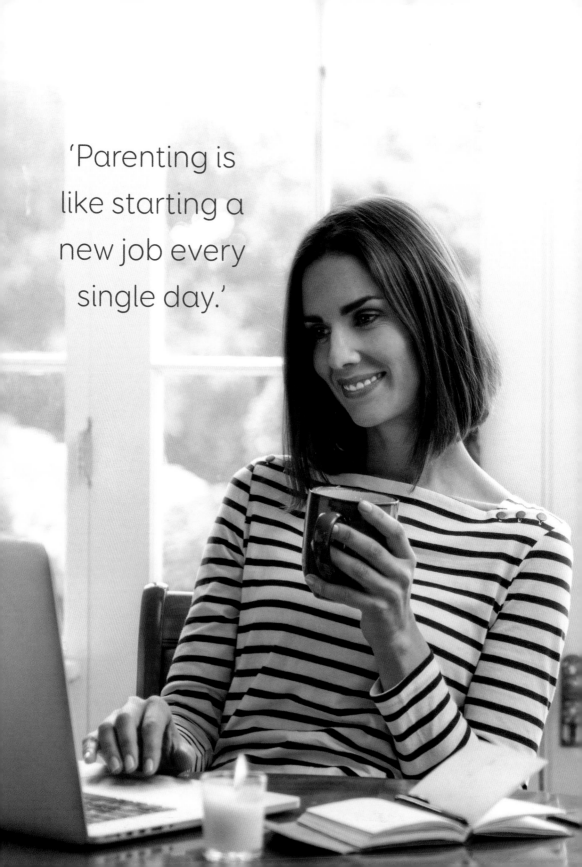

'Parenting is like starting a new job every single day.'

9

STRESS AND WORK/LIFE BALANCE

Stress is without doubt the biggest killer of our time. It can manifest itself in many ways and left unchecked can lead to serious illness. As a new mum it's easy to become stressed and indeed panicked about your newborn, your new life and your abilities as a new mum. The thing is that a little stress is good and necessary, so we are not looking to eliminate stress completely, but we do need to keep it in check and under control.

A certain amount of stress in everyday life is completely normal and we need it sometimes just to get things done. In fact, recent research has pointed towards stress strengthening the immune system and studies have also shown that it can protect against some diseases of aging, like Alzheimer's, by keeping the brain cells working at peak capacity. But as with anything in life, too much is bad for us. So again we are back to striking a balance, and finding your own individual balance is the key.

Personally, I need a certain amount of stress to get things done and it helps to motivate me. On the other hand, if I have too much stress I can't think, I get panicked and my world starts to

> **Today I'm going to relax. Oh wait, I'm a mom.**

crumble piece by piece. I used to get bad anxiety attacks because of stress, but I have learned to use various destressing techniques to prevent them from occurring. Hopefully these techniques will work for you, too.

As I have said before many times in this book, becoming a new mum can be overwhelming and it can also be very stressful. I found trying to leave the house stressful, in case I forgot anything the baby might need. I became worried about routines, feeding, development and so many other things. What I have learned is that when you are calm, that energy gets passed to your baby and indeed the rest of your family, almost like a domino effect.

Stress can present itself in so many ways:

* You can experience aches and pains all over your body and have digestive issues. The first place I notice stress is in my stomach. I used to develop really bad digestive issues from chronic stress, including once being hospitalised in Spain because I was so worried and stressed I couldn't go to the bathroom and my colon had become completely blocked. Our bodies will always show us signs of distress, but unfortunately we're not always listening.

* You can experience dizziness, nausea and palpitations and you can often be susceptible to illnesses as your immune system is weakened, leading you to pick up colds and bugs easier.

* You might start to notice you have a poor memory, more negative than positive thoughts and you can be worried and anxious a lot as you go about your day. (Use my Stop–Catch–Change tip on p.115.)

* Your appetite and eating habits can also be affected and you will often hear people say that they either can't eat or they overeat when they are stressed. I'm an overeater because I use food as a comfort when stressed, but both extremes are bad for your health.

* You'll often see people biting their nails or chain-smoking or indeed using alcohol or drugs to cope with stress, but these are all just temporary measures that will only make the situation worse in the long run. I know because I smoked heavily for nearly 18 years. Now, through my struggles with depression and anxiety, I know that the only way to cope with stress is to find some balance.

As a new mum you can feel moody, irritable and agitated, but above all you might just feel overwhelmed, isolated and lonely sometimes, especially in the early days. All of these feelings are completely normal, it's how you deal with them that makes the difference.

My favourite stress-busters

Stretching

A good stretch can help to release tension in your body. When we have a new baby, we can easily become stiff from carrying baby seats, buggies, etc. Your body might also be tense, especially in the early days when you are nervous and cautious with your little one. So a good stretch works wonders for your body. (See www. alisoncanavan.com for stretches you can do at home.)

Check in with yourself and breathe

An instant way to help calm yourself is to simply breathe. Watch and observe how your breath changes when you are stressed, sad, excited, nervous or indeed content and happy. No matter where you are and no matter what you are doing, you can always and instantly check in with yourself and breathe. It will calm you and help you to think clearer, enabling you to cope better in any situation.

Mindfulness and meditation

I absolutely love meditation and I practice every day. The power, and in my eyes magic, of meditation does not happen during your practice but outside your practice, in your everyday life. Regular practice helps you to cope with stress better, increases optimism, calms your nervous system and enhances your life in so many ways (see Chapter 8).

Routine

I fought against routine for such a long time, believing it wasn't for me and I didn't really need it. The truth is that we all need some routine and stability in our lives, especially when we have kids. I don't have a very strict routine, as my job is not nine to five, but as your kids grow you will start to notice that a routine of some sort is essential for the whole family. Kids actually thrive on it. The biggest thing I have noticed and realised over the past four years is that even though I still have many different jobs and I am currently back in college, structure and routine have enabled me to be much more successful, efficient and yes, you guessed it, less stressed! I have a morning and an evening routine I rarely stray from, which helps keep order in our crazy lives!

My very basic routine is like this:

I start each day with the words 'Thank you' as my feet hit the floor and then I breathe, stretch and have warm water and lemon. Then we have breakfast and get ready for school and work. I work from home, so as soon as I drop off James I do 15–20 minutes of yoga and meditate before starting my work day. If I have a meeting, I get up before James to do this.

In the evening, when I collect James, the golden rule is 'presence'. That is our time together. We have tea, homework, fun and storytime and then I get everything ready for the next day. As a mum this is a lifesaver because it saves stress and time in the morning and allows everything to run smoothly. So the night before I iron clothes, prepare lunch and write a list for the next day.

Adult colouring books

This is one of my more recent finds. I'll be honest, I absolutely love helping James colour on those kids' place mats in restaurants and I find it very relaxing, but my mum used to give out to me (yes, I'm a grown-up) as I'd to get annoyed when someone (anyone) coloured on my area. Now we all have our own colouring books and

I find it incredibly therapeutic. The adult books encourage you to focus and concentrate, which helps you practice mindfulness because you are so involved in the colouring you can't think about anything else. You'll be happy to know I have also learned to let James share with me and before you get carried away, no, he's not allowed to colour mine, instead we have a special book we do together! I find colouring helps me to keep focused and then I carry that focus into other things in my daily life. It puts me in a mindful, not 'mind-full', mood and helps to calm me.

Knitting and sewing

When I was in school we learned to knit and sew and I think they are really valuable tools for boys and girls because they are useful and incorporate mindfulness and relaxation. There are lots of great knitting clubs and people find them very therapeutic.

Exercise

Any and all exercise is a great stress-buster, so have fun with it and try new things. Sometimes all it takes is a walk to help make a dark day look brighter. Yoga is also amazing, as is Pilates, because you are working with your mind, body and spirit all at once.

Essential oils

My house is full of incense and essential oils. I love essential oils and I carry around some miniature-sized oils on my car keys, including blends called 'energise', 'serenity', 'calm', as well as some peppermint to help with my digestion as I struggle with certain foods at times. Essential oils are natural extracts from the seeds, stems, flowers, roots and bark of plants. But make sure you choose certified pure essential oils that are natural and therapeutic grade as these will provide you with the safest and most effective health benefits. Essential oils can be used aromatically to affect mood and open airways; topically for quick absorption into the body through the skin; and internally for immune and digestive support. (There's lots more information on this at www.alisoncanavan.com – search for 'essential health'.)

Healthy eating

Nothing fuels stress more than caffeine, cigarettes and alcohol and I know because I have used all of these things to excess. They are actually stimulants, so they will increase your stress rather than reduce it. So at the very least try to reduce all of these and replace them with water, herbal teas and fresh food. Avoid too many refined sugars and don't leave long gaps between meals.

Journal

This is by far my most powerful tool. It can help you to pinpoint your triggers and helps to release emotions and worries. Writing down your hopes and dreams, as well as what you are grateful for, helps you to focus on the positives, which in turn helps to reduce stress.

Affirmations

I am the queen of affirmations and if you see me walking down the road or driving in my car, you can be guaranteed I am repeating an affirmation to myself. I find them powerful and they have helped me to heal and focus. Here are my top 10 that I use regularly – and remember, they can be anything as long as they are positive. You can personalise them to your individual situation and day:

My top 10 stress affirmations

1. My mind is mine to control.
2. I can let go of my stress.
3. I am letting go of my worries.
4. I take time for me each day to help reduce stress.
5. As I relax, I free myself from stress.
6. I trust the present moment, knowing that it is the only thing I can control.
7. Obstacles and challenges help me to grow.
8. I take a breath when life gets crazy.
9. I am relaxed and free from stress.
10. I can find balance in my life.

Sleep

Although hard to come by in the early days of parenting, sleep is vitally important so whenever you can, grab a nap.

Dancing and singing

Yes, dancing and singing can be done anytime and anywhere and have the ability to change your mood and an atmosphere almost instantly. If I feel my day is getting off to a bad start, I crank up the music and dance. If I'm sitting in the car getting anxious and restless, I turn up the tunes and sing and chair-dance (safely, of course). You can dance with your baby and as your baby grows you can enjoy nightly or morning discos, just for five minutes a day. This will help to lift your mood, it gets your body moving and very simply music gives us the ability to express our feelings and emotions. For me, music is therapy, whether I'm happy or sad. It allows me to release and let go. You might feel silly for the first minute, but with good music, you'll soon forget that and just get into the groove!

Learn to say no

This is one of the hardest but most important things you can do as a new mum for yourself and your family.

I was the yes kid and to be honest, I'm still working hard on this. I was terrified of saying no because I didn't want people to dislike me, I didn't want to disappoint people and, if I'm brutally honest, I have a terrible fear of conflict. What I soon learned, however, was that when I actually had to say no, when I had become ill from spreading myself too thin, some people became annoyed anyway.

You can't please everyone all the time and I often feel a part of us is conditioned to say 'yes'. We have to say yes to our parents and teachers as we are growing up, so very often when we start a new job we feel we have to say yes all the time to our bosses and colleagues, and this naturally filters into all areas of our life.

When you are a new mum, you need to prioritise and the people who matter will understand. When someone asks for your time, especially in the early days, don't answer straightaway: first, think it through; then weigh up your priorities and see if you genuinely have the time.

Then, if you want to say no, say it by way of a thank you (practising gratitude) first, and then politely decline. For example:

1. I really appreciate the invite, but I'm just focusing on family time and the baby at the moment.
2. Sorry I won't be able to make it, but thanks for thinking of me.
3. Honestly thank you for the invite, but I'm just too tired.
4. Thanks for the invite, if it wasn't so soon after the baby I would love to go, but hopefully we can get together soon.
5. Thanks for asking and as soon as I have settled into a routine, we'll be in touch.
6. I'd love to do this, but right now I just don't have the time.

So the lesson here is that you can say 'No' and be polite about it. The people who matter will understand and saying no will increase your productivity, confidence and stress levels in the long run.

As your baby grows and eventually goes to school, you will face lots of different challenges in this area as a mum. For example, when they start school you have to find a balance between mothering, school activities, helping others out and playdates and if you are a working mum, throw that in there too. So it's really important that you never say yes on the spot because you might regret it later. I find I need to look at my week and try to balance it out. If I agree to help someone out on a Tuesday evening and someone asks for help on Thursday too, I need to make sure I am dividing my time fairly between work, home and what I call 'community duties' for my family; in my opinion, family must come first.

Always consider the length of time you are committing. I have been caught out on this in the past because a lot of the time my jobs take a lot of preparatory work and if I fail to factor that into my planning, it leads to difficulties in successfully juggling work/college and being a mum. Just remember, if you have too much on your plate you are no good to anyone, most of all yourself and your family.

So that's quite a long list of stress-busting ideas and I hope some of them resonate with you and fit in with your lifestyle. I find it's a combination of the above that works for me. But please don't feel overwhelmed by this list as I don't do everything every day. Instead, I try to tune in and listen to what I need. I don't always get it right, but I'll never give up trying and that is what's most important in this life because we are all on a journey where we are constantly learning and growing, which keeps us on our toes if nothing else.

Work/Life balance

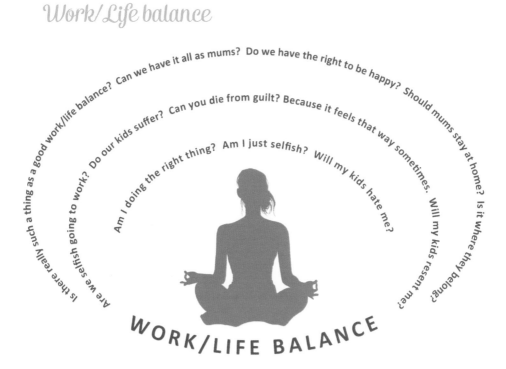

Is there really such a thing as a good work/life balance? Can we have it all as mums? Do we have the right to be happy? Should mums stay at home? Is it where they belong? Will my kids resent me? Are we selfish going to work? Do our kids suffer? Can you die from guilt? Because it feels that way sometimes. Am I doing the right thing? Am I just selfish? Will my kids hate me?

WORK/LIFE BALANCE

The reason I started this section with all those questions is because I have received a variety of e-mails and comments after radio and television interviews from mums with very, very strong views on this topic. Well, I also have a very, very strong view on this topic, which is do what's right for you!

That's right, do exactly what's right for you and not what's right for your sister or your best friend, and definitely don't do what society thinks you should do because you'll end up miserable.

Let me make one thing very clear before I continue: all mums are working mums. Staying at home is actually the most difficult job in the world. It's constant and you don't even get a lunch break most days! That is why I think the best thing a mum can do is reserve judgement and offer support. If you want to stay at home, then do that; if you want to go to work, or have to, you should be able to do that without feeling guilty. A good way to figure this out is to write a list of pros and cons and then a list of things that you feel you can't change but would like to. This will give you a great starting point that will realistically show you where you are and the options available to you.

For example, I knew I couldn't model forever and I had been back to college a ridiculous amount of times over the years in an effort to figure out what I was going to do next. I completed all my courses but after each one I knew that it was not what I wanted to do. This is not necessarily a bad thing, even though at the time I thought it was the end of the world and that I was never going to find my purpose in life.

When I became a mum I pushed through my fears and tried new things. I decided to go back to college because once I had done out my list of pros and cons I was sure that the investment would be worth it down the road, even though there would be sacrifices in the meantime. My main focus has always been James and after that I would fit in work, college, writing, etc., often staying up late at night and getting up very early in the morning to complete work. People often ask me how I do it, but I know it's not forever and that I am laying down the groundwork for our future. Following your dreams and taking risks is definitely not the most comfortable or the easiest way to do things, but in the end it's worth it.

The reason I am sharing my story is because when you become a mum, something shifts. Your priorities and interests can change and, contrary to popular belief, this part of your life is the beginning of a very exciting new chapter.

As a new mum you might want to:

* give up work and stay at home;

* quit your job and start a new career;

* go back to your old job;

* take extended maternity leave;

* start your own business from home;

* go back to college and follow your dreams or up-skill.

What's important to know is that it is possible to choose any of these and make it work for you. That's not saying it will be easy. As a working mum, some months I barely break-even and some people ask me is it worth sacrificing time with my son when I'm barely making ends meet. I never focus on the negative. My answer is that I love my job and I am much happier working and pursuing a career than being at home.

Your life does not end when you have children – in fact, a whole new world of opportunity awaits. Don't get me wrong, you have extra responsibility and less time to achieve what you want to achieve, but if you are doing something you love (we'll come to that later), you can be happy doing both. I believe that you can have everything, just not all at the same time. You will have to sacrifice different things at different stages, yes, but don't ever give up on your dreams.

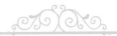

A Happy Mum = Happy Children

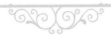

THE END

I cannot tell you how true and how important this very short story is and you need to know this and believe this as a new mum. So figure out what is right for you and your family. There are a lot of things you might not be able to change for now, like a job you hate, for example, but I'll share some tips that will hopefully help you in that regard.

Deciding to return to work

Taking the decision to return to work can be daunting, especially if you have had a long gap on your CV. You'll be nervous entering the world of work again and that's okay and completely normal. My advice would be to approach a new job like you approach parenting: give it everything you've got!

As your kids grow you might feel like you're ready to head back to work – they don't need you as much and have started school and it's understandable to want to do something for yourself. You might want to start your own business from home or start a blog about your interests and passions in life. A lot of women like to have their own income as it makes them feel independent and they miss it when it's gone. Some mums just like the headspace of being out of the house. There are other ways to achieve this, of course, such as volunteering for a charity in your community.

We go through different phases in our lives and what fulfils us today might not fulfil us tomorrow. As the years go by you might want to try something new or you might just have a burning desire to go back to work. The point is that we are all different and how you feel is how you feel, so follow your feelings.

It's normal to be scared when you go back to work, get a new job or indeed start your own business. I was terrified the first week I sent my column in to the editor of *VIP magazine*. You feel like you are opening yourself up, and of course you are, but you have to because otherwise you wouldn't progress.

When you're feeling daunted or lacking in confidence, always think to yourself: what's the worst that can happen? They don't like it or they say no. Well, that's okay, that's manageable, I'll just have to move on to the next one.

I have had far more people say No than Yes in my career. I spent over half my life in castings being told No. Since I became a mum, I can't tell you how many people have said No. I have spent countless hours on presentations that have been turned down. I started a couple of businesses that failed. I have had e-mails gone unanswered and meetings that have simply just not gone my way. In fact, I have been told No so many times, I am now more driven than ever. In other words, what we might perceive as failures and knock-backs can be blessings in disguise.

So keep trying, and don't get disheartened. If you don't know what you want to do, keep trying new things until you find something that ignites a passion in you. There is nothing more rewarding in life than doing something you love. If not in work, then choose a hobby you love. There is always a way!

Going back to work after maternity leave

The first thing I would say to all new mums is to simplify your life as much as possible. We all think everyone else is coping better than us, but the reality is that most mums struggle to get any balance into their lives, never mind getting it right.

Before you start to beat yourself up and feel guilty about the decisions you make, know and accept that there is no right or wrong way to live. There is only the way that you want to live and hopefully that is a way that helps you to feel content.

Returning to work isn't always straightforward. It can throw up all sorts of emotions – some of the ones listed below might resonate with you.

* As a new mum, you will probably feel like your confidence has taken a blow.

* You might feel unsure as to whether your colleagues will look at you in the same way.

* You can feel nervous about your ability to step back into your role.

* You might be feeling anxious and guilty about leaving the baby.

* You might feel like you are just not good enough.

Let's face it, you've spent the past few months gurgling, changing nappies and covered in sick and now you have to jump into your professional mode again, which can be very daunting.

Top tips to get work-ready

* Keep in touch with work colleagues and ask them to keep you informed of any major changes at work. This way you won't feel completely out of the loop when you return. Meet work friends before you return and refresh yourself with what is going on.

* Get organised: this is the most important one for me. You need to create lists and make them your best friend. Whether you have lists on the wall or in your phone, they will help to keep you focused. And is there anything more satisfying than checking things off a list? Set alarms on your phone if you are busy and tend to forget things (perfectly normal for mums!).

* Don't underestimate the power of having everything prepared the night before, including your own clothes. If I have a lot to bring I pack the car the night before, which means my mornings are less stressful for everyone. Leave spare everything with your childcare of choice, clothes, nappies, wipes, food and toys. I used to buy inexpensive clothes and leave them there in case of an accident/emergency.

* Pre-plan your meals for the week. Make your baby food in batches and freeze and do the same for your own dinners. Switch to Internet shopping as it cuts time and you can do it from the comfort of your own home when the baby or kids are asleep.

* If you are struggling to stay on top of the cleaning and washing, ask for help. If you can afford it, get someone in to help for a few hours a week. This will help to ease the pressure. I send my large items to the cleaners sometimes when I am really busy and it is sheer bliss when they come back ironed and folded.

Nearly every day at work people ask me: how do you do it? When I get to work I switch to professional mode and leave my stresses at home. But the truth is, I struggle so much when **trying to balance work and home life.** I need to take jobs whenever they come in, which means that one week I'm incredibly busy and the next I have nothing on. On empty weeks, my panic levels can shoot up for financial reasons. This sort of stress is pointless as it changes nothing and only succeeds in making me unhappy.

There are definitely a few things you can do that can help this situation.

Top tips to balance work and home life

* **Keep a list** and schedule five minutes of 'me time' every day. This can be as simple as sitting down with a cup of tea on your own and taking a few long deep breaths.

* **Get the kids involved** in chores from an early age and help them to understand that a sense of responsibility is very important. Children need to realise that there are no magic wands, but I also do my best to make chores fun. We have a race to see who can put the most toys away first. James also helps me to hang out the washing and he loves emptying the dishwasher, which is actually one job I would rather he didn't do as it's costing me a fortune in cups and plates!

* **Make sure you are getting some form of regular exercise** as this will keep your mind clear and help you cope better. Going for a short walk every day as a family can be great for all of you and you'll be surprised at how much fun it is. Most of the time we dismiss these ideas because we 'don't have enough time'. I'm sure we can all find 10 minutes every day,

and 10 minutes a day is 70 minutes of quality time for the whole family each week. I remember a mum telling me to lower my expectations of myself. I was shocked at the time, but now I completely get where she was coming from. This simply means that unless you're superwoman, you can't have the washing, ironing, cleaning, cooking and school runs done and work full-time. Believe me, trying to do that could actually make you sick.

* **Try not to talk too much about the baby at work:** it's so tempting to constantly talk about the baby, but what I realised is that most people don't care, so keep your work life professional (unless you are asked about the baby) and your home life separate. Save the gushy talk time for your friends and family.

* **Choose childcare that suits you and your family:** if you have relatives or a grandparent who's happy to help, that's great. Alternatively, you might decide to choose a childminder, au pair or a crèche/daycare facility. You need to feel comfortable and confident that your child is being taken care of and is happy while you are at work. Don't be afraid to ask questions, do your research and talk to other parents

to get some first-hand advice about local childcare facilities. I chose James' crèche, The Toddler Inn, based on great referrals, low staff turnover, my instinct and the fresh nutritious food they serve every day. Ask your childminder to send you updates and photos in the early days so you don't feel like you are missing out. Expect both of you to cry in the early days. I found this part the hardest to cope with because I used to feel awful driving away. As time went on and if James was upset, I used to hang around and check back in. I was always reassured when he was laughing and having fun.

* Quit feeling guilty: of course, this is easier said than done, but there is no scientific evidence to suggest that children are harmed when their mums go to work. The reality is that most families need two incomes these days just to make ends meet, but be assured that once your kids are in a loving, caring environment, The American Academy of Pediatrics reports that they will thrive, regardless of whether or not the mother works outside the home, as long as they are well loved and well cared for. Some mums even find that they are better working either full- or part-time as they feel fulfiled and are therefore happier.

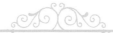

Rebuild your confidence

C- Care for yourself

O- Organise your day

N- No negative thoughts about yourself

F- Free yourself from the judgement of others

I- Identify your needs and goals and work towards them

D- Deal with your emotions

E- Explore your talents and passions

N- Nurture your soul with mindfulness/meditation

C- Completely trust your instincts

E- Easy does it – Rome wasn't built in a day.

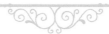

It is possible for us all to build up our confidence at any time. I find journaling helps me to focus on the positives and distil my goals clearly for myself. Try writing down five of your greatest achievements in work pre-baby and then also write down five things you would like to achieve. That will give you something concrete to work towards and help you focus.

What if I am unhappy in my job?

If you have got to work and you dislike your job or you just don't want to work, try to make the best of it. If you really hate your job, remember that you are doing it to give your family the best life that you can.

A lot of mums would rather be part-time or in a different job, but instead of focusing on what you don't have, try cherishing the time you do have when you are home in the evenings. Also, during your work day use your lunch hour to do something you enjoy: take a class, meditate, colour, meet a friend, exercise, relax or go for a walk on your own, which can be blissful. Sometimes you have got to make your own fun and happiness, even in the midst of a less than ideal situation.

My best back-to-work affirmations

1. If I did it before, I can do it again.
2. I choose progress over perfection.
3. I feel confident in my abilities to return to work.
4. I'm strong and ready and I can do this.
5. I am an inspiring role model for my child/children.

The Golden Rule of achieving a work/life balance: be present when you are with your kids

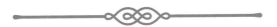

My golden rule, which I picked up from parent/child relationship expert Joanna Fortune, is 'presence over presents'. She said this on a parenting course I attended years ago and it hit home instantly. How many of us buy presents and material goods to make-up for not being around or as an apology to people? Your time is the most important gift you can give your children. The very best family memories we have relate to time we spent with our parents, not of presents we received. I lost my dad 16 years ago and I remember time, not things – the tumble I used to do on his legs or the twirling in the garden and how he used to throw us all up in the air and laugh with us. Those are the things that make me feel loved and make me smile to remember them. So make your time with your children really count. Put down your phone, focus on your child and have fun. There is no better cuddle than the cuddle when you return from work each day – after all, they are the reason you get up and do what you do.

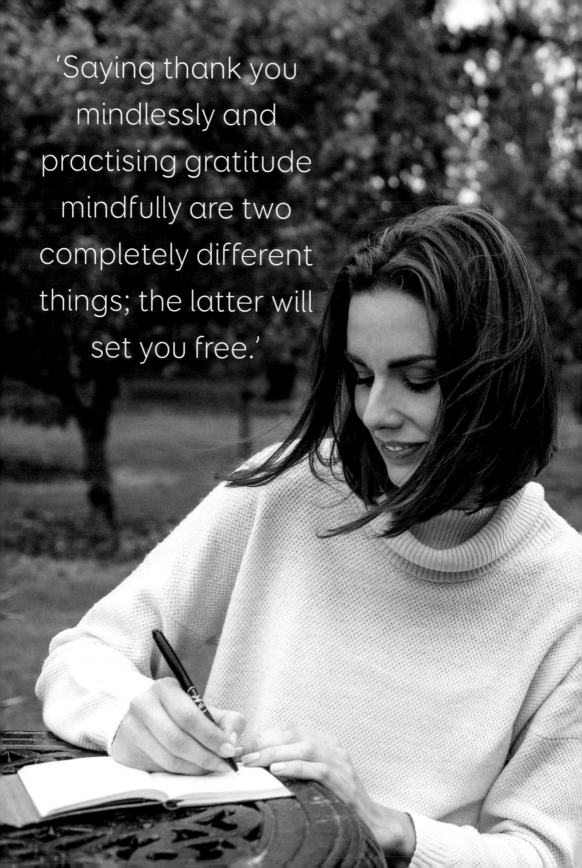

'Saying thank you mindlessly and practising gratitude mindfully are two completely different things; the latter will set you free.'

THE ART AND THE IMPORTANCE OF GRATITUDE

Gratitude works both ways: it's the art of giving and receiving. I have always been interested in the body, mind and spirit connection from a very early age, but because I was so preoccupied trying to find things outside myself to fill voids, the whole idea of what gratitude really meant eluded me. The energy of gratitude is like no other and although I was never ungrateful, I never really felt gratitude deep down inside, acknowledged it and lived it. As an adult living in this crazy world I was always worried about tomorrow and next week. I had forgotten about the beauty and simplicity that surrounded me in everyday life.

I relearned all of this through my son. Having a child was like a rebirth for me into this world. Once again I got an opportunity to appreciate the beauty in all things, big and small. The first time James saw a flower, his wonder at an ant crawling and the first time he saw an airplane flying through the air he said *Wow*, and I did too. I began to think differently, to see differently and I began to get excited about each day: What would happen? Who would I meet? What would I see?

My change was gradual, but as I changed, I shed my old skin and grew quite comfortably into my new skin. I will admit that at first it felt like it wasn't going to fit, but when you are on the right path you will fit beautifully into yourself, just the way it was meant to be.

For so long we have been taught that eating well and exercising is enough to keep us healthy, but it's simply not true. As our body, mind and spirit are one and not separate entities, we need to nourish all of them equally. This is why being grateful and practicing some form of mindfulness and meditation (see Chapter 8) is so important to complement good food and exercise. It all interconnects: the food we eat nourishes our body and mind; exercise increases endorphins to help mood as well as getting our bodies moving and keeping them healthy; meditation and mindfulness help us to be present in the world; and gratitude is the magic that ties it all together.

Let's just think about the words *Thank you* for a moment. How many times a day do you say it. As basic manners go, it's one of the first things we teach our children. 'Now what's the magic word, James?' I often hear myself say. We have come so far with our manners in this house. It started off with 'peas', aka Please, and 'danku', aka Thank you. Throughout the toddler years it was 'Danks', usually with James' chin stuck to his chest because he didn't want to say it but had to, especially to strangers! 'Chinitis', as I call it, is when your toddler is going through the tantrum or 'No' phase and their chin seems to get stuck to their chest. This is usually accompanied by a lower lip sticking out and a sad face, but they grow out of this too and funnily enough, like most things, you'll miss it when it's gone.

But as we grow up we begin to get mixed messages about gratitude. As children we can be labelled as ungrateful and as the saying goes, if you hear something often enough, you start to believe it. Instead of telling children they are ungrateful, we should be teaching them to be grateful for what they have. We throw these words around, not really understanding the strength of their meaning. When we hear negative things about ourselves, we start to feel like we are not worthy and this is when we move away from feeling truly grateful to just saying Thank you for the sake of it, because it's good manners.

What does gratitude do?

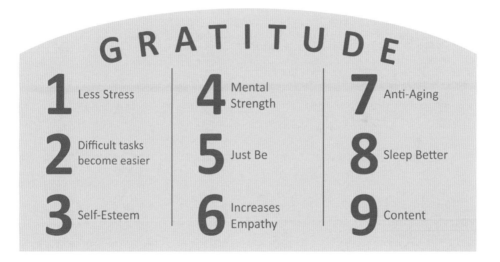

GRATITUDE

1 Less Stress

2 Difficult tasks become easier

3 Self-Esteem

4 Mental Strength

5 Just Be

6 Increases Empathy

7 Anti-Aging

8 Sleep Better

9 Content

We are all seeking the same things in life: we want to know that we matter and we want to belong. When you become a new mum, sometimes you can feel lost in the world. You spend so much time on the baby that you forget who you are and what you like and what makes you happy. It doesn't have to be this way.

When you start to practice gratitude, the universe listens and difficult tasks become easier. You will be able to cope better and what mum doesn't want that! Everything in your life will become more vibrant and colourful and you will really start to feel like you're living. You will start to see more and more coincidences happening in your day-to-day life and what you expect will start to show up for you.

Gratitude awakens our true sense of self and this is really important because we all have so many different personas. For myself, I have work Ali, mum Ali, friend Ali, daughter Ali, sister Ali and so on, and I never knew which one was the real me. But when all those faces slip away, the real me is what's left: the non-judgemental, compassionate self. Deepak Chopra puts it elegantly: 'The true self, once discovered, is the source of creativity, intelligence and personal growth. The true self is the basis for being deeply optimistic about how life turns out and who you really are, behind the screen of doubt and confusion.'

Believe me, once I changed how I saw the world, the universe started showing me so many signs that I was on the right path and making the right choices. I would randomly bump into strangers and a conversation would start and that conversation would be exactly what I needed at the time. This began to excite me and this excitement is contagious. My friends and family wanted a piece of it too and that's the thing, anyone can have it! I stopped attracting negative people, which was something I was pretty good at. For a while, when I started to change how I lived, I felt quite isolated and lonely as the phone never rang, but after a while I realised that it was the best thing that ever happened. Old, authentic friends showed up and I met wonderful new people and my circle became supportive and positive, which is the only circle you want and need.

As a new mum I was forced to work on myself because I felt lost, and because of that work I found the real me. Don't get me wrong, this is an ongoing process and it will be a lifetime's work, so don't expect to wake up one day and be happy and perfect. Let's leave that to Hollywood, please! But at least I now know that I'm on the right path and, more importantly, enjoying the journey rather than just trying to get to the destination.

I accept my failures and there have been many these past few years, but now I'm not afraid to fail anymore. You will constantly question your abilities as a new mum and there will be nights you will question if you made the right decisions and did the right things. This is all normal and part of being a parent, but gratitude will help you see what you are doing right, which in turn will give you confidence. We all need reassurance as parents because there is no manual for life – we are all making it up as we go along.

The most important lesson I learned was that gratitude turns what we have into enough. You will never be happy with anything you want unless you are happy with what you have right now. This is powerful and challenging because we are brought up in a world of want and need. There is always something you don't have but need to buy, or the ideal body you want but don't have right now. I wanted a happy family with a few kids and I'm a single mum with one little boy. It's not what I ordered, but I'm so happy my order was switched up somewhere along the way and every day when we wake up both James and I say *Thank you* as we put both feet on the floor.

For me, gratitude turned denial into acceptance and confusion into clarity because it is a catalyst for real change in your life. It helps you to shift from a negative to a positive state of mind. Listening to negativity and being negative is exhausting. Being grateful helps to ground you in the present moment. Life has become so complicated and we are all so stressed and worried. Try to look at gratitude as your anchor and no matter what size your ship is, it will help you to regain control and steer your life in the right direction.

This is really important for new mums because you can start to feel like you have no time for anything but the baby. As you are human, you may also start to feel resentful and mourn for your old life. You might feel that having a baby is turning out to be a very different experience from what you thought it would be. You're wrecked, your boobs are saggy and your bum is in the wrong place. These are just a couple of examples of how negativity can start to creep in and take over, and this is also why a gratitude list is incredibly important, especially when you are having a bad day.

I remember chatting (moaning) to a friend on the phone one day and I said I couldn't think of one thing to write on my gratitude list that day. Somewhat impatiently she said, 'Just write that you woke up'. That moment was a huge turning-point for me and a really important lesson that there is always something to be grateful for.

Setting intentions and writing a gratitude list

In my daily life gratitude and intentions work side-by-side. At the beginning of the week I set my intentions for the week and then every day I have goals or intentions for what I want to achieve that day. This might seem like a lot of work, but it takes no more than

5–10 minutes a day, so 35–70 minutes a week. Not bad considering there are 168 hours in the week!

I have a gratitude diary and I write down 10 things that I am grateful for every day and why I'm grateful for them. The lady who helped me with my post-natal depression first advised me to do this, and it really helps. It shifts your focus from negative to positive and you start to see all the things that you have instead of what you don't have.

Every night I hold my gratitude stone (read *The Magic* by Rhonda Byrne if this idea is new to you) and list all the things I'm grateful for that day; I often challenge myself to see how many I can list. I'm really a child at heart and I find this exercise fun! I also get James to do this and it's wonderful to see how many things he is grateful for. There is a really special spiritual place in the west of Ireland called Dzogchen Beara and I have spent some time there on retreat, writing and for personal healing. The spiritual director is Sogyal Rinpoche who wrote *The Tibetan Book of Living and Dying*, which is a book that helped me to make some sense of death when I lost my Dad. As this place means so much to me, I kept a small stone from the meditation garden and it sits on my bedside locker and it is the stone I hold every night. So choose a small stone from somewhere you love – it can be a beach, a garden, the zoo or anywhere that has meaning for you. If the stone means something to you, it will become priceless and magic!

> "There is always something to be grateful for."

I used to set intentions in my head, but I soon learned that the only way they worked for me was to:

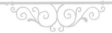

say it – write it – do it – reflect on it

I find that we are all full of great intentions,
but we need to actually follow through to
feel good about ourselves.

It can be absolutely anything that you need to cross off your
To Do list, but you can also have long-term intentions and goals,
such as: buying a new house; going back to college; changing jobs;
healing family rifts; living a healthier lifestyle; saving for a holiday;
saving for a new car; see my favourite band in concert next year, etc.

1 JANUARY
An example of an intention list for a new mum:
I am going to get some exercise
I am going to eat well
I am going to practise self-care
I am going to ask for help
I am going to accept help
Today I'm going to live in the present
Today I'm going to have fun!
Today I'm going to call my friend back
Today I'm going to be kinder to myself

I would also make a list of all your intentions and desires for the coming year on New Year's Eve or, if you prefer, make a vision board. I made my first vision board as a young model and pretty much all of it came true. Sometimes people find it easier to see pictures and visualise their future that way. I used to cut pictures out of magazines and quotes and make them into my story or the story I wanted. Again, be warned, this is so much fun!

Here's an example of a gratitude list:

I'm grateful for my son
I'm grateful for my home
I'm grateful for my family and friends
I'm grateful for my health
I'm grateful the sun is shining today

I usually develop mine into something a little more detailed, like this.

I'm so grateful to be healthy because for a long time I wasn't and today I have the energy and vitality to live life to the fullest.
I'm so grateful for my son, who teaches me about love and life everyday.
I'm grateful for my journey up till now because each and every second has taught me a valuable lesson.
I'm grateful for my happiness and I never take it for granted.
I'm grateful for my job and that I work at something I love.
I'm grateful for my home because it's filled with laughter and love.
I'm grateful to wake up to a new day because every day is an opportunity to start again.

I'm so grateful to be surrounded by friends and family who love me
unconditionally.
I'm truly grateful for new friends and new opportunities.
I'm so grateful that I'm a mum because it is the best job
I've ever had.

. You can also pass on the gift of gratitude to those you care about. Set a challenge and ask them to write a gratitude list or have a gratitude quiz and ask family members what they are grateful for. This will get gratitude flowing and if people feel and see the benefit, they will continue.

How will you know it's working?

Very simply, you will notice that you start to see things differently. You will feel more connected to yourself and feel more contented and happy. You will start to show up for yourself more in your own life, to take responsibility for your own happiness and people will start to show up for you. The greatest obstacle for most of us in life is ourselves: so get out of your own way.

I find writing a gratitude list helps me to push through my fears. We all have fears and while it's okay to be scared, real growth takes place when we take baby steps and work through these moments. You will know it's working when you do things that you would never have dreamed about doing before.

I also found that by practicing gratitude I stopped rushing mindlessly through life. When that happened, I was shocked at how much more life I had time for, and believe me I'm an incredibly busy person so this is a miracle.

As a mum you will start to see that the best moments always come after a struggle, especially in the early days.

> *Be your own hero and believe in yourself, and have the courage to simply show up for yourself in your own life.*

Do you remember in the chapter on nutrition (Chapter 5) I said that when you eat good food it is like delivering a very special parcel or present to yourself? And your cells, those little messengers, are super-excited and simply can't wait to open their gifts? Well, the same applies to gratitude. Grateful thoughts also act like little messengers, delivering messages of joy to your cells, and they start having a positivity party inside you!

I know it's easy to feel grateful when life is going well and I also know that not every day is like that. Most days you will experience ups and downs and the same goes for your journey into parenting. But one thing I do know is that in life we all need to let our light shine brightly and be proud of it. So be proud and grateful for who you are. You are the author of your own book and you can start a new chapter whenever you like. To quote Albert Einstein:

> *'There are only two ways to live your life. One is as though nothing is a miracle. The other is as though everything is a miracle.'*

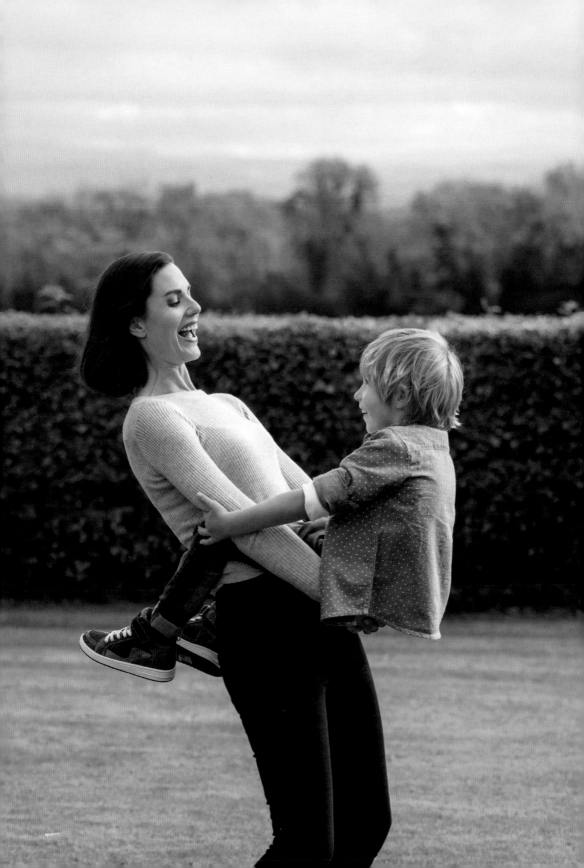

EPILOGUE
AND THE STORY
GOES ON ...

When you become a mum, things will never be the same again – they will be better. It's so easy to get caught up in the negatives and become worried and anxious about doing things right. The most important part of parenting is to enjoy it. Sometimes we are so flustered as mums that we miss truly magical moments. In the early days, sit and simply watch your baby, let time stand still and tell yourself how proud you are because you did this and you are amazing.

As your baby grows, savour the wonder of their development: the first smile, when they sit up, start holding things, their first words and, of course, the excitement of their first steps. It really does go by too quickly. James started school last year and although a lot has happened in that time, it seems he is growing up too fast. I have jokingly asked him to stop growing; he says he can't help it, but promises he'll never leave me. As a mum I would love that to be true, but I know James will grow up into a young man and live his own life.

There are a few things I want for both of us, but the most important one is great memories of happy times. I want him to remember a mum who had fun and gave him time, not things. I'm often asked if we can have it all as mums, and I do believe we can, just not all at the same time. You need to ask yourself: what is important right now? Choices, not sacrifices, will have to be made and be careful how you view them. Make peace with your choices and with yourself as a mum.

Throughout this book I have touched on various ways that you can try to help to either restore or find balance in your life. I do believe we all need to find our own individual formula. Some people are very lucky to get away with poor lifestyle choices for a long time, but it all catches up with us eventually. I spent my life taking short-cuts and I won't lie, making positive life changes was hard in the beginning because I still had to convince myself I wasn't missing out on the old days. What I have come to realise is that the past is the past and life changes every second and every hour of every day and resisting that change will only make things harder.

I did not introduce all the changes at once, but rather in small bite-size chunks over time. If you make small changes and stick with them, they will become habit. I don't have to think about meditating or writing a gratitude journal anymore as they are as natural as eating and sleeping for me, but it did take time to reach that point. You need to find your own formula and your own passions and if you are struggling and want to find something outside of parenting that you are interested in or good at, just keep trying and don't give up.

I cannot tell you how many classrooms I have sat in knowing that afterwards I would have to ring my mum and tell her, 'Sorry, this is not for me'. I never thought I would find my purpose in life. Yet as it turned out, it was during my darkest days, when I could see no future or light, that just over the hill, out of sight, my brightest days were waiting.

So to all the wonderful mums out there: love yourself with all your heart, take risks and follow your dreams. Don't fall into the trap of the 'being a mum means I can't' excuse. During my pregnancy so many people told me my life was over, that I would never travel again, that my career would end. Your life is not over when you become a mum. Your priorities shift and you will have a period of readjustment, but you are still the same person you were before.

My greatest teacher is my son. He has taught me how to live and I have pushed myself harder than ever before because of him. My life didn't end when I became a mum, in fact, it's only just begun.

A WORD OF THANKS

This book has been a journey that would not have been possible without the help and support of so many people. First of all, I would like to thank Avril Mulcahy who introduced me to Deirdre Nolan from Gill Books, who in turn sat patiently with me for hours in The Westbury Hotel and listened to my vision for *Minding Mum*. To the incredible team at Gill Books, your support, guidance and encouragement has been essential for me to push through some difficult writing days, but we did it. So a huge thank you to Sarah Liddy, Catherine Gough, Rachel Pierce, Claire McVeigh, Teresa Daly and Emma Lynam.

To my amazing Mum, who has always supported and loved me unconditionally. When we lost Dad, you dedicated your life to us. I want to take this moment to let you know how deeply appreciated you are. Thank you for being a great Nana and always being there for James and for me, especially during my illness or when I'm working away on my dreams.

To my sister Jennifer and her husband Myles, I love you dearly and thank you for helping me to take that first step on the ladder to rebuilding my life. My middle sister Laura and her husband Ronan, thank you for your neverending support, encouragement, hope and vision for better days ahead. To the babies (not anymore!), Grace and Kate. You will always be my baby sisters. Thank you for all your love and support.

To my cousin Rita Connaughton, who has been my Earth angel. To David Gilna, if you didn't believe in me so much, there would probably be no book to read today. To Andrea Hayes and Caroline Grace Cassidy who have always supported me.

To Rebecca Morgan, I love you more than words can say. Thank you for always listening. You have been much more than an agent and your support has carried me through some very difficult times. To Pamela Duffy, Aifric Hyland and Karen Clince, there is no way there would be a book without all of you. Your support, endless hours of babysitting, food deliveries, accounts and picking up James allowed me to finish chapters and, eventually, a book!

To John Fitzpatrick for always being there for me and being a wonderful godfather to James. To Noel and Mary Sutton. To my grandparents Maureen and Tommy Canavan, I love you both dearly. My uncles Noel, Francis, Aidan and their families. Andrea Casey, Jenni Crawford, Aideen O'Neill, Donna Ward, Bree Cullen and Louise O'Connor. The Mannions. Sadie and Paddy Cowan. Elaine Prendeville and Michael O'Doherty for giving me a chance, and *The Evening Herald* for printing my first ever article on mental health. Paul Henderson, Sebastian Hamilton and colleagues in the *Daily Mail*, especially Linda Maher and Lynne Sharman, thank you. My trainer Siobhan Byrne at BodyByrne. To Caroline Jackman. To Dylan Townsend for really understanding me and being a great friend. Caroline Murphy for a lifetime of friendship. Claire

Heaslip for your help and support. Dr Carly Walsh for helping me with my research and fact-checking. Zarah and Andre from www.cherishme.ie. The team at Honda Ireland. Emma Buckley & Amy Buckeridge for your endless love and support. To Des Canning and John Lahart. To my Aunty June, I miss and love you.

To the entire team at Spirevision. Thank you so much to Donie Dickson and to Edina for understanding my vision and for your patience, your love and your neverending support; also to Dave Rooney for work on the website.

As a proud ambassador of Walk in my Shoes and as mental health is an important chapter in this book, I would like to thank all the staff at St Patrick's Mental Health Services, including CEO Paul Gilligan for reading through some of my work; my fellow ambassadors Brent Pope and Adam Clayton, thank you both for all your support. A huge thank you to Madge Fogarty from PND.ie who spent hours on the phone to me when I was very sick.

Thank you to Stephan Terrass, who is a visionary in the world of nutritional supplements and who cares enough to make clean products that work. A special thanks to Olive from PPC Galway for helping me with the omega section in this book. To Richard Burton from the Irish Institute of Nutrition and Health (IINH) for all your support and help with the nutrition chapter. Thanks also to Dr Ashok Varadkar and his wife Miriam.

My obstetrician, Dr Hugh O'Connor, and the most amazing midwife in the world, Katherine Quinn. To Dr Edmond O'Flaherty, thank you from the bottom of my heart for finally getting to the root cause of my problems. Your combined practice of nutrient therapy and allopathic medicine is changing and saving lives every day. Your diagnosis has helped me to live a life that is now anxiety- and depression-free.

To my spiritual home, Dzogchen Beara in west Cork, thank you to all the staff, and especially to Malcolm MacClancy for your generosity and kindness.

Thank you to Ryan Tubridy, who dealt with such a sensitive issue (PND) so well on *The Late Late Show* back in 2011. I was so nervous about telling my story but that night changed my life for the better in so many ways, so thank you.

To everyone who has touched my life through the years, to all my agents, including Andrea Roche, Joanne Byrne and all the team at Presence PR, fellow co-workers, models and friends, thank you all.

There is not enough room in this book for all the things I want to say to those who have been so essential in my life, so I have written a longer thank you on my website: www.alisoncanavan. com. I hope you all know how special you are to me.

Photo shoot credits

All clothes from: Oasis, Warehouse, Karen Millen, H&M, Mothercare, www.graceandaibell.com.
Make-up: Derrick Carberry (Callanberry), Ann Marie Carey.
Make-up for photo on p.212 by Virginie at www.CouleurCaramel.ie.
Hair: Jenni Crawford, Kazumi Hair Salon.
Photography: Spirevision Studio.
Illustrations: Sean Branigan from www.storyboardworkshop.com.
Main photography: Edina Valentova, assisted by Juraj Jabionka.
Locations: Phepotstown House; Spirevision Studio.
Food and extras: Pearse Healy/Feena McCormack.
Video on my website to accompany the shoot was shot by: Evan Henegan and Mary Walsh of http://ieweddingvideos.ie.